DIET

ENLIGHTENMENT

THE REAL SECRET TO WEIGHT LOSS

RACHEL L. PIRES

Published by Diet Enlightenment
www.dietenlightenment.com
Published in the United States of America

ISBN: 978-0-692-90821-1

DEDICATION

This book is dedicated to my husband for all your love and support, and to my parents for always believing in me.

CONTENTS

INTRODUCTION

To the mind that is still, the whole universe
surrenders.

—Lao Tzu

I am not a licensed nutritionist or physician, and
this book is not intended to replace nutritional
counseling, but it is a dieting philosophy based on my
personal beliefs and experiences. I set out to write this
book because I found what I like to refer to as diet
enlightenment. I'm truly grateful for this blessing and
wanted to share this knowledge with anyone who has
ever struggled with weight loss. I hope this book makes
you laugh, gives you strength and inspiration, helps you
reach your dream weight, and most importantly helps
you find peace with dieting.

CHAPTER 1
THE ELUSIVE DIET

I have not failed. I've just found 10,000 ways
that won't work.

—Thomas A. Edison

If it feels like you've tried ten thousand diets, yet
weight loss still eludes you—you're not alone. In
fact, most dieters fail to lose weight or keep the weight
off long-term. But why is that? After all, weight loss is
an exact science. It's an interesting paradox to consider.
Despite what a billion-dollar dieting industry wants
you to believe, there is a secret to losing weight and it is
far simpler than you've imagined.

So, what is this great secret? Surprisingly, you
probably already know about it; however, might have
forgotten during your struggles with dieting over the
years. Are you ready for it? Weight loss is all about
calories, *calories* and *calories*. It's not about fat, not about
protein, and not about carbohydrates. I'm not saying
that these things don't matter, but I have found that
successful weight loss has always been and will always
be about consuming fewer calories than you burn.

You can go on the cookie diet, the caveman diet, the
only-eat-with-chopsticks diet, or even the vampire diet.

That was a little humor for you! But in all seriousness, it doesn't matter which diet you choose because as long as you stick to it and end up consuming fewer calories as a result, you will lose weight. Okay, so this isn't exactly esoteric knowledge, but still most dieters overlook this fundamental formula when it comes to weight loss. After years of being conditioned by the dieting industry, it's no surprise that most individuals are genuinely confused and struggle with how to lose weight.

Now I'm not a doctor, although after all the time I've invested, I feel like I should have a PhD in it—the D standing for dieting. Nevertheless, after years of experimenting with different diets, I am overjoyed to say that I have finally become awakened or what I like to call achieved diet enlightenment. Today, at 5'2" and 105 pounds, I weigh the exact amount I have always wanted to, and I maintain it easily. Most importantly, I have found true peace with dieting. Surprisingly, the secret to successful weight loss was far easier to understand and implement than I ever thought.

On my journey to diet enlightenment, one of the surprising lessons I learned was that you can lose weight initially on almost any program that you stick to. Not what you were expecting to hear? This means that diet programs such as Weight Watchers, Jenny Craig, Nutrisystem, Atkins, and the South Beach Diet will all help you lose weight.

Now, you might be wondering why diets with different methodologies all work. Well, despite the fact that they have different rules and systems, every single one of these diets if followed religiously will result in the consumption of fewer calories at the end of the day. Think about it; how come one diet allows you to eat bread and pasta, while the other one declares the end to carbs? I promise you, it's not the gimmicks that are working here; it's the calorie deficit they result in.

While most diets will work at first, keeping the weight off long-term is a different story. Haven't you noticed that the majority of people who lose weight end up putting it back on later? Do the majority of dieters just happen to lack self-control? I don't think so. I honestly believe that most diets are just not built for long-term use and weight-loss maintenance.

For example, if you lose weight on a strict low-carb diet, but you love carbs, you'll gain the weight back when you return to your old eating habits. Or if you lose weight based on eliminating certain foods, when you ultimately start incorporating them, you'll likely put the weight back on. You see weight loss programs that aren't built around calorie counting can work short-term, but they usually don't work long-term.

The key is to lose weight eating the types of food you love, so when it comes time to maintain it, the only difference is that you're getting more calories. While you can lose weight on almost any diet, I have found that there is only one true method for weight loss that will keep the weight off permanently and easily— and that is monitoring your calories with your own customized plan.

When I finally achieved diet enlightenment, one of the things I realized was that there are a lot of false perceptions about how to lose weight. Despite the fact that there are likely thousands of books and websites dedicated to the topic, most people still generally find the concept of dieting abstruse. That's why I titled this chapter the elusive diet. Weight loss is really quite simple, but the dieting industry has created a lot of confusion about how to lose weight. Honestly, with all the contradictory information available, it's no wonder that most people find themselves lost.

Some of the diets out there are outright dangerous and others are healthy, but expensive. Some diets claim you have to avoid certain foods, others claim you have to eat certain foods, and yet still others claim you have to eat certain foods at certain times of the day. Now, eating certain foods at certain times of the day may or may not be advantageous to your health. You'd have to speak to a nutritionist about that one. But as far as weight loss goes, in my experience, these gimmicks are a bunch of baloney. And not even the delicious kind!

Any seasoned dieter can relate to the frustrations that accompany the typical diet. One of my friends once pointed out that the word "diet" includes the word "die" in it. At first we laughed considering the irony, but then we realized that for the majority of people, that is essentially the experience they have with dieting. Most dieters nearly starve themselves or eat such a bland diet that they are practically dying existentially.

That is no way to live! I'm here to tell you that dieting does not need to cause suffering, stress, boredom, or even depression. And it certainly does not need to mean a lack of tasty food. In fact, my whole philosophy on dieting is that it can and should be easy, enjoyable, and rewarding. As you will learn later on in this book, if you are not eating food you like and not feeling satisfied throughout the day, then you are doing something wrong—and you will not have long-term success.

I'm sure you know by now that the weight-loss industry is a multibillion-dollar industry. New fad diets come out all the time and are immensely profitable. Think about how many ridiculous diet products you see each year, but people continue to spend money and there continues to be a demand. I included some pretty silly dieting examples earlier to make you laugh, but also to make you think. Many of the fad diets out there claim to offer quick results, but are dangerous and inherently built for long-term failure. In fact, it's failure after failure that keeps the dieting industry so lucrative.

In actuality, the concept of weight loss is really quite simple and painless. No, I'm not a crazy person. You see with the right approach, you'll find you can eat the foods you love and never be hungry, and have weight loss that feels effortless. Folks, I am not selling a magic carpet here. I'm just reminding you of what you always knew—that weight loss is all about the calories.

Out of the commercial diets out there, I think there are a few good ones that don't ignore the importance of calories. The Weight Watchers program, for example, is essentially a calorie counting diet that converts the calorics to a system of numbers called points. It incorporates fat and fiber into the calculation, which is great for your health, but not a necessity for weight loss. While I think it's one of the best commercial diets, my question for you is—do you really need to spend all that money when you could have easily achieved the same results on your own? While I have nothing but positive things to say about Weight Watchers, I have found that you can count your calories just as easily as you can count your points—actually it's even easier.

Don't get me wrong, many of the commercial diets out there are good and if you stick to them you will lose weight; however, I want to show you that you don't need them to succeed. You can do it on your own for free. All of the tools that you need to lose weight are available to you at no cost, except for the food itself that is. Also, think about all the money you will save and all the new outfits you can buy! You could spend hundreds or even thousands of dollars over a lifetime on diet programs, or you can just do it yourself—all you need is the right information!

In this book, we are going to explore the science of calorie reduction, but also how to get the most out of the calories you are consuming. Get more bang for your buck that is, or for your calorie! We're also going to redefine your relationship with food and dieting, and show you how most diets actually work against your body's natural tendencies. You may not have realized it, but you can truly lose weight easily and effectively while eating the food you love.

You mean no more eating rice cakes or frozen meals? No more counting the minutes to lunchtime? That's right—you don't need to try so hard when you're eating food you genuinely like and you're watching your waistline shrink. No one ever said you're supposed to be hungry or eat boring meals while on a diet. It doesn't matter if you need to lose five pounds or a hundred pounds; the science of weight loss is all the same.

I struggled for years with dieting before I finally came across this approach to weight loss. While you may have written off calorie counting in the past, you will be shocked to see how quickly you lose the weight when you apply the techniques in this book. You too can be the skinny girl or guy at the party, fit into your old jeans from high school, or finally lose those last few pounds. You can stop obsessing about weight loss and start concentrating on the important things in life. If you stick to the guidelines outlined in this book, your struggle and obsession with dieting and keeping the weight off will be a thing of the past.

CHAPTER 2

THE MULTIBILLION-DOLLAR DIETING INDUSTRY

Insanity is doing the same thing over and over again, but expecting different results.

—Rita Mae Brown

T hink of all the money you've invested in weight-loss books, services, products, meals, or supplements—yet are you still struggling to lose weight? Or perhaps you know of someone who seems to have tried everything; nevertheless, they still can't keep the weight off. It's like that old adage that says, "If you always do what you've always done, you'll always get what you've always got."

Well, it's time to stop trying the same old things and start thinking outside of the box. This is where diet enlightenment can help. But, before we explore the enlightened approach for how to lose weight and keep it off, let's discuss this multibillion-dollar dieting industry and clear some of the smoke and mirrors.

Each year, Americans spend billions of dollars on weight loss; yet, over two-thirds of the country remains overweight or obese. According to studies conducted by researchers at Harvard University and Imperial

College London, thirty-four percent of Americans are obese, another thirty-four percent are overweight, and only thirty-two percent are at a healthy weight.[1] That's sixty-eight percent of the country that needs to go on a diet!

According to a study published in the American Journal of Preventitive Medicine, it was projected that by the year 2030, 42 percent of U.S. adults could be obese.[2]

Holy smokes, I guess it is a good time to start investing in the weight loss industry. And yes, for the companies that sell diet products and services, it'll continue to be a very lucrative business. Face it, when you fail to lose weight or lose weight but gain it back, companies will profit.

The unique thing about your typical dieter is that even after multiple failed diets, they are almost always willing to come back for more. And, when faced with failure, they usually don't blame the diet; rather they blame themselves for lacking willpower and determination. It's quite a convenient scenario for the dieting companies. Maybe it's just a coincidence that many of the popular diets today promise dramatic weight loss, but don't offer long-term results. I'm not trying to say it's a conspiracy here, but I do find the overall situation intriguing.

Despite billions of dollars spent on weight loss, sixty-eight percent of Americans remain overweight and obese, and the dieting industry continues to grow. Yeah sure, blame it on a lack of willpower, a lazier generation, overly processed foods, or the increasing presence of larger portions and fast food restaurants, but I don't entirely buy that rationalization. Despite these realities, I believe that the dieting industry is also greatly to blame.

Years of misleading information, contradictory dieting methods, unrealistic plans, and false expectations have muddled up the facts and led many dieters to believe that weight loss is difficult and confusing. And yet at the same time, companies sell "magic bullets" for weight loss with persuasive advertising. I know it takes a bit of naivety for some of these gimmicks, but you have to consider that some dieters are willing to try anything—often at any cost. Taking advantage of customers is nothing new to big business. Think about it, if weight loss and maintenance were easy, it just wouldn't be as profitable.

Have you ever stopped to think about why there are so many different types of diets and approaches? It's not like the secret to weight loss is a mystery and scientists are still trying to crack the formula. If you were to do research in any of the top medical journals or resources, you'd find all the knowledge you need to lose weight.

For example, research from the *New England Journal of Medicine* cites that reduced-calorie diets result in clinically meaningful weight loss regardless of which macronutrients they emphasize; and the possible advantages for weight loss from a diet that emphasizes protein, fat, or carbohydrates have not been established.[3] What this means is that when it comes to weight loss, it's not about fat, not about protein, and not about carbohydrates—it all comes down to the calories.

Still, show me a room full of dieters, and I guarantee you that at least half of them are on some type of low-carbohydrate program. While the research is out there in medicals journals and publications, most people are distracted by the dieting propaganda that is ubiquitous in today's society. And while there are good diets and information available, there is also a whole industry worth of misleading information.

Trying to navigate dieting in today's society can be downright confusing for just about anyone. Even many celebrities with disposable incomes and resources still have the same frustrations with weight loss. Look at Oprah for example. She's a smart, successful, and inspirational woman, yet her ideal weight still eludes her. What does that tell you? It's not about time and it's not about money. You don't need to hire a dietician, a personal trainer, or even an annoying assistant to follow you around all day. Even the most driven and determined people can struggle with weight loss without the right knowledge.

It doesn't matter how many diets you've tried because with the wrong approach, you could spend your entire life struggling with weight loss and never master it. On the other hand, it doesn't matter what your age, gender, or net worth is because with the right method you can have astonishing success. It's all about dieting efficiently. However, for the majority of people who don't know better, the business of dieting will continue to be a puzzling and precarious task.

Losing weight and staying thin has become one of the great desires for women in today's society. Despite what was considered the epitome of attractiveness in the 1950s, models have been getting thinner and thinner. Haven't you heard the saying "You can never be too rich or too thin?" At the heart of this trend is a multibillion-dollar fashion industry. This industry has often been at the center of controversy for promoting eating disorders and unrealistic expectations.

If you look at high-fashion models on the runways or in magazines, they are typically tall, extraordinarily thin, and often have boyish figures. Ironically, if you were to ask most men, the majority doesn't find the emaciated look attractive. Rather, they prefer women who are slim, toned, and with curves in the right places. There is a difference between being thin and having a healthy BMI versus being clinically underweight and emaciated.

While I think all sorts of shapes and sizes are beautiful, the problem with promoting the runway-model look is that the majority of women can never live up to these ideals of attractiveness. And for those who can, it's sometimes at the risk of their health or in extreme cases their life. Think about it, if you're never too thin, there will always be a reason to lose weight.

Over the years, as both men and women sought to get thinner, many creative and interesting diets emerged. One of the most popular and yet questionable dieting trends to arise in the past few decades is the anti or low-carbohydrate craze. It's fitting—since that's what I find these types of diets, crazy! Now don't get me wrong, limited carbohydrate plans like the Atkins Diet or South Beach Diet will work when followed properly and can help you lose weight. However, I want to share with you the real reason why I think these types of diets work.

Please keep in mind that the following comments are based on my personal opinion. Since I'm not a doctor, I'm not going to question the effects that low carbohydrate or high protein diets have on the body; however, I strongly believe that diets that restrict certain types of food only work because you end up consuming fewer calories in the process. Contrary to popular opinion, too many carbohydrates will not make you fat, but too many calories will. Regardless of the gimmick, I seriously believe that any diet that works, only does so because it results in fewer calories consumed.

In 2004, an episode of the BBC science program *Horizon* investigated the effectiveness and dangers of the Atkins Diet. The theory behind Dr. Atkins' diet was that by restricting starchy foods like bread and pasta, and eating mainly proteins and fats like meat and eggs, you could eat as much as you want and still lose weight. Dr. Atkins' claimed that on his diet you would actually burn more calories than usual. He believed you burn more calories when your body uses fats and proteins as fuel, and could lose unused calories during the process known as ketosis.[4]

According to *Horizon*'s investigation of this claim, neither of these explanations was found true.[5] The findings confirmed what I suspected all along—when followed correctly the Atkins diet is effective, but only because you end up consuming fewer calories. Nevertheless, this investigation brought some interesting details to light.

Per this research, one study found that without apparently trying, people on the Atkins Diet were eating less than they normally would. It seemed that eating large amounts of protein could act like an appetite suppressant and somewhat turn off hunger—essentially making people want to eat less calories.

If the research indicates that foods high in protein can help control hunger, then we can incorporate this knowledge into our food choices. We will touch upon this concept in a later chapter. However, despite the latent benefits of protein, I still don't recommend converting to a purely low-carb, high protein diet for a number of reasons.

As the study suggests, we don't have any evidence on the long-term effects of diets high in protein and low in carbohydrates. The American Dietetic Association (ADA) believes that individuals who stick to high fat, high-protein and low-carb diets may be setting themselves up for health problems in the future.[6] Most doctors suggest that the healthiest diet for your heart is one high in grains, vegetables, and fruit, and low in salt and animal-based products. Honestly, I'm not sure where the truth lies regarding the dangers of high-protein diets. After all, this book is not about how to eat healthy, it's about how to lose weight.

But personally, I'm not willing to take the potential health risks of a long-term high-protein, low-carbohydrate diet. It just doesn't seem natural to me. Plus, even if eating insane amounts of protein would completely curb my appetite, I'm not willing to cut out the food I like, especially when I know that I can lose weight just the same while eating a balanced diet. I'm also a big believer that when you make a specific food forbidden, it just makes it even more attractive.

It's important to understand that people's tastes vary. What might work well for one person, might be torture for another. A low-carb, high-protein diet could work well for you. But if you're like most people and prefer a balance, then it's not the right program for the long-term. You can lose weight just as easily by monitoring your calories.

I happen to love bread and pasta, and I eat a lot of both, yet I still always lose weight when I follow my calorie guidelines. Contrary to what my grandmother used to say, bread doesn't make you fat , too many calories makes you fat. Regardless of what I eat, I gain weight when I eat more calories and lose weight when I eat less.

Think about it—the majority of thin people aren't running around only eating meat. If that were the case, then we might have an argument here. But, it just isn't so. Plenty of individuals lose weight and easily maintain it through calorie and portion control; they don't need to cut their carbs to do it and neither do you!

While it seems the jury is still out on the dangers of low-carb diets, the most dangerous plans are the fad or gimmick diets. You can spot these diets from a mile away. They sound like, "Lose twenty pounds in ten days," or "Drink this mysterious liquid and drop ten pounds in a day." These diets sound too good to be true because they are.

Don't be fooled. Unless you are seriously overweight, your body can only lose one to three pounds per week at a healthy rate. Anything more is likely water weight. These types of diets prey on the wallets of despairing dieters, but what's worse is that they can be downright dangerous.

According to the article "The World's Most Dangerous Diets," a few of the most dangerous diets of all-time include: the Master Cleanse, the Sleeping Beauty Diet, the Grapefruit Diet, the Tapeworm Diet, and the Cotton Ball Diet.[7] I'm sorry, but if your diet plan encourages you to sleep all day to avoid food or ingest dangerous parasites to lose weight, it's time to reevaluate your priorities.

There are another two mind-boggling diets that have recently gained popularity. The first one is called the HCG Diet, which combines drops or injections of HCG, a pregnancy hormone, with just five hundred calories a day.[8] I hate to break it to you, but you don't need HCG to lose weight on five hundred calories a day; that's called starvation.

The second diet is called the K-E Diet and is becoming particularly popular with brides-to-be. On this diet, individuals have a feeding tube inserted into their nose that runs to their stomach and are fed a constant slow drop of eight hundred calories a day. This diet promises that over ten days, the regimen can lead to about twenty pounds of weight loss, or about ten percent of a patient's total weight.[9]

Not only are extreme low-calorie diets dangerous for a multitude of reasons, but I'm curious to know how much of that weight loss is attributed to muscle mass and water. Plus, why would anyone resort to something so radical, especially when you can just as easily lose weight by watching your calories? I think it comes down to the fact that some dieters are so desperate for progress; they are willing to try anything to get the weight off. But the problem is that not only are these extreme diets dangerous, they won't keep the weight off long-term. What's the point of losing weight, if you're just going to gain it back?

Diet pills are another one of those "magic bullet" solutions that are appealing to many who will go to any length to become thin. Diet pills suppress the appetite, which causes you to eat less. However, diet pills can have really dangerous side effects, and they are only a temporary fix. Also think about this—unless you're planning to stay on diet pills for the rest of your life, when you finally go off of them you'll most likely gain the weight right back because you haven't learned how to manage hunger the right way.

Instead of pursuing diet pills and other gimmicks, you need to learn how to eat smarter, so weight loss isn't so arduous. Besides why go to such dangerous lengths when you can easily achieve the same full feeling by just changing the way you eat. You don't need any of these tricks to get down to your dream weight. It's so much simpler than that.

Now that we've discussed many of the dangerous diets to avoid, I'd like to discuss some of the good ones, the really effective weight loss programs that don't deny the importance of calorie counting. As I've mentioned before, I think Weight Watchers is one of the best commercial diets out there. It seems to be one of the only programs that gives you the flexibility to eat what you want, while still monitoring your caloric intake or points. But you should note that it's really just an adaptation of calorie counting and some great marketing.

Weight Watchers takes the calorie counting formula one step further by incorporating fat and fiber into its system. Now they are correct in the sense that too much fat can be bad for your health and may make you feel hungrier, and bumping up fiber is good for you and can help you feel fuller. But at the end of the day, it really is only the calories that affect your weight. If you don't feel like spending the cash to get the Weight Watchers proprietary formula, you can always just count your calories for free!

Diets such as Nutrisystem and Jenny Craig also rely on calorie restriction and portion control too, but with a bit of a different approach. They offer prepared meals that have been separated into categories, so you don't need to track your calories—they've already done all the work for you. While these types of programs are convenient, easy-to-follow, and very effective, I do have one major concern. You haven't learned how to research, measure, count, and prepare on your own. You run the risk of gaining the weight back after you stop eating their meals.

I think it's important to learn the skills that come with researching the calories in food, measuring your portions, and recording what you eat. If you choose to pursue a diet program with prepackaged meals and stick to it, you can definitely lose weight. Just make sure you're able to switch to your own calorie counting or portion-control plan once you've stopped eating the prepared meals, so you don't gain the weight back.

All in all, the dieting industry really is a mixed bag. There are good diets out there based on sound scientific research, but the industry is also wrought with misleading, unrealistic, and dangerous information. You can't rely on the dieting industry to have your best interest at heart. As an enlightened dieter, it is very important to understand that the dieting industry is foremost a business.

You can lose weight with a commercial diet, or you can lose weight completely on your own using the techniques in this book. The choice is up to you. Personally, I'm a big believer of *why have someone else do for you what you can do for yourself.* As Thomas Edison once said, "If we did all the things we are capable of, we would literally astound ourselves." By the end of this book, you'll learn everything you need to know to lose weight and keep it off permanently.

Remember, regardless of what you might hear, the only proven way to lose weight is to consume fewer calories than you burn. My friends, it doesn't matter if you're eating low carb or high carb; vegetarian or animal-protein; or six times a day or twice a day—it has always been and will always be all about the calories.

CHAPTER 3

WHY EATING HEALTHY WON'T NECESSARILY MAKE YOU THIN

Common sense is not so common.

—Voltaire

E ating healthy can do amazing things for your mind and body. I believe the right food can make your brain operate more efficiently, enhance your mood, boost your immune system, improve your physical appearance, and deliver a great amount of natural energy. Also, what you choose to eat can influence your blood sugar, raise your insulin level, and affect your body in many ways. It can even be argued that food is the most powerful drug we put into our bodies. It is undeniable, the significance and effects that food has on us. However, despite all of these benefits and what may seem like common sense, choosing to eat healthier will not necessarily make you thin.

One of the most common dieting myths or misconceptions is that simply by eating healthier, you will lose weight. While this may seem like sensible logic, the reality is that eating healthy will not guarantee weight loss. In fact, you don't even need to eat healthy to lose weight. Now don't get me wrong, I am not encouraging individuals to avoid healthy choices when trying to lose weight. In fact, I am one of the biggest proponents of healthy eating. The healthier choices you make, the better you will feel. The better you feel, the easier it will be to stick to your plan. However, becoming enlightened as it refers to dieting, is about discovering the truth.

One of the fundamental truths of diet enlightenment is that calories don't discriminate. A calorie is a calorie regardless of whether it is considered healthy or unhealthy. Since it's entirely possible to gain weight while eating healthy and lose weight while eating unhealthy, you can't rely on conventional wisdom. That's why my personal philosophy is to eat healthy for your health, but to eat the right amount of calories for your waistline.

Now you might be thinking—what about the general population? Since for the most part, the healthier eaters are skinnier than the junk food eaters. That's because healthier eaters are often more cognizant of what they put into their bodies, and typically healthier food is lower in calories. However, I know plenty of thin people who are junk-food eaters and plenty of so-called healthy meals that are packed with calories.

Think about this; cucumbers are low in calories, but avocados are not. Watermelon is low in calories, but raisins are not. Red wine vinegar dressing is low in calories, but olive oil certainly isn't. Not all healthy foods are created equal when it comes to calories. And while healthier food is typically lower in calories than unhealthy food, it's not always the case. You just can't assume when it comes to calories.

Did you know that there are more calories in a half cup of almonds than in a full-size Baby Ruth candy bar? Or that you could basically eat five ice cream sandwiches for the same amount of calories found in two cups of granola. Quick, someone better call the ice-cream man!

At one of my neighborhood restaurants, Romano's Macaroni Grill, the seemingly healthier Parmesan-crusted Sole has more calories than the Fettuccini Alfredo. If you go to California Pizza Kitchen, the Waldorf Chicken Salad has more calories than the Four Cheese Ravioli! At Bertucci's Italian Restaurant, the Roasted Eggplant Pomodoro has more calories than the Baked Tortellini with Chicken Gratinati. In what universe do we live in, in which a fish, salad, or even vegetable dish has more calories than pasta with cheese or cream sauce! But in these cases, it's true.

Don't get me wrong; overall healthy food is still usually lower in calories than unhealthy food—but my point is you just can't assume that healthy means low calorie. You might be shocked to find that some of the healthy or so-called low-fat diet foods are actually very high in calories. That's why if you want to lose weight, you need to be mindful of your calories.

It concerns me to hear individuals say that they want to lose weight, so they are just going to eat healthier. That's great and they are definitely on the right path, as long as they are also monitoring their calorie intake in some way. One family friend of mine was trying to lose thirty pounds before her wedding, and she said that she was just going to eat healthier because she didn't believe in calorie counting. While I normally don't like to meddle, I didn't want to see her disappointed on her big day.

I quickly but nicely pointed out that the Starbucks Blueberry Muffin she had eaten for breakfast had almost double the calories of a Krispy Kreme donut, and the large California Pizza Kitchen salad she was currently consuming had dressing and toppings on it that could have equaled two McDonald's Big Macs. In fact, we hadn't even gotten to dinner yet, and she had already consumed over 1,500 calories without even realizing it. That certainly opened her eyes!

Now, my friend thought she was making the smarter choice by choosing what she thought was healthier; a muffin over a donut or bagel, and perhaps a salad over a few slices of pizza. While in most scenarios she would probably be right, in these cases she wasn't. Her mistake wasn't in trying to eat healthy, or in going to Starbucks or California Pizza Kitchen. In fact, I'm a big fan and frequenter of both since they make their nutritional information available online. Rather, her mistake was in guessing. See the thing about dieting is you just can't guess especially when it comes to calories.

This type of approach and thinking doesn't surprise me though. We've been conditioned to believe that weight loss is completely tied to eating healthy. You're familiar with this type of rationalization—order the veggie-burger instead of the hamburger, choose yogurt instead of ice cream, or perhaps grab a handful of nuts instead of chips. It seems healthier; it must be better for my diet!

Now, it's perfectly fine to make the healthier choice, but make sure you are doing it for the right reason. Choosing to eat healthy may help you prevent illness and live longer, improve mental performance and focus, give you more energy, and significantly improve your physical appearance. So choose to eat healthy for one of the abundant reasons why eating healthy is good for you, not because you have to for your diet—because you don't.

I hate to admit this, but in actuality, if you consumed the right amount of calories you could lose weight eating fast food for breakfast and candy for dinner; albeit, you would be hungry and end up pretty sick. You could also gain weight eating nothing but organic food. The bottom line is that you need to be cognizant of the calories you eat, regardless of whether they are deemed healthy or unhealthy.

Plus, eating healthy can have different definitions for different people. For some, it's about remembering to incorporate enough fruits and vegetables, or cutting down on foods that contribute to cholesterol and heart disease—although the causes often seem to be changing. For others, it's about following a vegetarian or vegan liftestyle. Yet for others, it's about eating real foods, avoiding overly processed foods, and focusing on organic and Non-GMO ingredients. How healthy or unhealthy you want to eat and how you want to define that, is really up to you. That's the beauty of this program—you can choose whatever foods you want based on your personal goals.

For those of you who are interested in eating as healthy as possible while monitoring your calories, you should note that according to a February 2013 study from the *New England Journal of Medicine*, the healthiest eating style appears to be the Mediterranean diet. The research shows that this style of eating reduces the risk of heart disease and overall cardiovascular mortality.[10]

The Mediterranean diet characterizes the traditional cooking style of countries bordering the Mediterranean Sea. It focuses on fruits, vegetables, whole grains, legumes, and nuts. It also recommends replacing butter with healthy fats such as olive oil and canola oil; and recommends using herbs and spices instead of salt to flavor foods. In addition, it limits red meat to a few times per month, and recommends eating fish and poultry at least twice a week. And yes, it does recommend drinking red wine in moderation.[11]

Now next year, this diet recommendation may be out and something else may be in. Again, what you choose to eat is completely up to you. When it comes to eating healthy, I like to focus on what I should eat instead of what I should avoid. I have found that when you try and eliminate foods entirely it just makes you want them more. Instead, if you focus on what foods you want to incorporate for health reasons, it's easier.

Ultimately, I try to eat healthy, but I don't put anything off limits and I don't drive myself crazy over it. For example, you might see me eating wheat pasta for lunch, but white rice in my sushi for dinner. Or, you might see me eating organic chicken one day, but a

Subway sandwich another day. I've even been caught eating grilled chicken , broccoli , and Doritos in the same day. To some that might seem silly, but I don't believe in all or nothing . I think it's more realistic to have a balance and give yourself flexibility.

Besides if you are going to stick to this eating philosophy long-term, it has to be something you can live with. Remember, this book isn't about how to eat healthy, it is about how to lose weight. Technically, you can eat anything you want and as long as you stick to your calorie guidelines, you will lose weight. While eating healthy is an important piece of the puzzle, it won't make you skinny unless you also watch those calories. My guess is that if you are going to all this effort, you don't want to try and lose weight, you want guaranteed results.

Overall you'll notice that the better you eat, the better you will feel physically and mentally, and that makes weight loss easier. Plus, as you'll learn about in chapter 8, many of the foods that can give you a lot more bang for your calorie are actually very healthy. But, perfection doesn't exist. It's nice to know that if you happen to eat something you deem unhealthy, you don't have to worry; instead just adjust your calories for the rest of the day and no harm done. That's one of the reasons I think this dieting philosophy works so well because it offers the flexibility and freedom to choose whatever food you want.

Seriously, I eat healthy most of the time, but sometimes a girl just needs to have a brownie sundae.

It's nice to know that you can have one once in awhile without sabotaging your diet! Remember, eat healthy for your health, but count those calories for your waistline.

CHAPTER 4

THE SKINNY ON
DIET AND EXERCISE

To keep the body in good health is a duty,
otherwise we shall not be able to keep our mind
strong and clear.

—Buddha

S imilar to eating healthy, exercise can do amazing
things for your mind and body. Working out can
help you burn extra calories, significantly improve your
health, and completely transform your body. However,
one thing exercise will not do by itself is make you thin.
According to the *TIME Magazine* article, "Why
Exercise Won't Make You Thin,"one of the most widely
accepted and commonly repeated assumptions in our
culture is that if you exercise, you will lose weight. But,
recent studies have found that exercise just isn't that
important when it comes to weight loss.[12]

It's a surprising but fundamental truth of diet
enlightenment that exercise is not a necessity for weight
loss. However, just because it isn't necessary, doesn't
mean I'm not going to encourage it. I have found that
exercise is very much like eating healthy; you don't
need to do it to lose weight, but if you choose to, you'll

look better, feel better, and find weight loss easier. But before we discuss the various benefits of working out, let's first explore the relationship between exercise and weight loss.

The fitness industry, like the dieting industry, is a multibillion-dollar business. Each year, Americans spend billions of dollars on exercise-related services and products. According to *Medical News Today*, some eighty percent of gym memberships are rarely or never used.[13] Talk about a profitable business model! Even for those who do make it to the gym, workout at home, or do other physical activities, many still find themselves struggling to lose the weight and keep it off.

For some time now, researchers have been finding that people who exercise don't necessarily lose weight.[14] Yet, many people still choose to disregard their diet and focus solely on exercise. Don't get me wrong—working out does burn calories, but it's just generally not enough to create the calorie deficit required to lose weight. Think about it, even if you were to work out five hours a day, if you still consumed more calories than you burned, you wouldn't lose weight.

I have found that one of the biggest problems when it comes to weight loss and exercise is that most people underestimate the calories they eat and overestimate the calories they burn. Unless you are a professional athlete, you are probably not working out to the extent where you can eat 5,000 calories a day and maintain your weight. And for those who are not monitoring their calories and just relying on exercise to lose weight, it's often in vain.

I once had this coworker who used to jog every morning and teach spinning class four times a week, but despite all that time logging workouts, she was still on the chubby side. That's because while she worked out way more than I did, she didn't monitor her caloric intake. On the other hand, I knew someone who lost seventy pounds through the Nutrisystem diet without any exercise. Funny enough, after he lost the weight, he started exercising like crazy and has never looked better.

Either extreme isn't good, but it's important to understand how weight loss works, and that it is not dependent on working out. The truth is that you can lose weight with diet and exercise, or you can lose weight with diet alone, but you'll be hard pressed to get results just with exercise.

Many people think that working out gives them a free ticket to eat as much as they want. I see it all the time. Someone walks out of the gym or an exercise class and then rewards him or herself with a high-calorie meal thinking that it won't count. Research shows that there is really no such thing as the "after burn" effect.[15] Even if you do a great workout, if you then go and eat 2,000 calories for dinner, you're still eating an additional 2,000 calories. You can definitely workout and add additional calories to your diet, but it might not be as many as you'd think.

If you really want to see how many calories you burn for a workout, you can get a reliable approximation by using the Calories Burned Activity Calculator at www.freedieting.com/tools/calories_burned.htm This is a free resource that gives you an estimated calculation based on your gender, age, height, weight, and duration and intensity of the workout. There are many similar resources available online that use these characteristics to help you more accurately determine how many calories you burned.

And if you're not sure how many calories you burned, it's always better to underestimate. If you find that you're watching your diet and eating your exercise calories, but still not losing weight, there is a high likelihood that you're overestimating your workout calories.

Even though we've established that exercise is not necessary for weight loss, I still recommend it because the benefits of exercise are immense. Not only can it help you burn extra calories, but exercise can also improve your heart health, decrease your blood pressure, help prevent dementia, and give you lots of natural energy. Exercise can improve your mood and give you extra motivation to stick to your goal. But beyond all the advantages to your health, there is one additional benefit that you might find pretty compelling.

Did you know that you could literally transform your body through weight lifting and the right exercises? You can effectively reshape your entire physique. For women, I'm not talking about bodybuilder muscles here. I am talking about getting toned! You know, getting rid of those pesky bingo arms and upper thigh saddlebags. I mean who needs a plastic surgeon when you can transform your body naturally? With the right weight lifting and exercises, you can essentially give yourself a breast lift, reshape your derrière, or create the illusion of an hourglass figure. With the right combination of diet and exercise, you can drastically improve your figure.

Have you ever seen women who are skinny, but somehow still look flabby? That's because they lack muscle tone. You want to look thin and healthy, not thin and sick. Whether your preferred body type is model Adriana Lima, actress Sofia Vergara, musical artist Beyonce, or professional wrestler Nikki Bella, they all have one thing in common—they are in shape and they have beautifully toned bodies. Regardless of what the fashion industry might say, I'm telling you; slim and curvy, toned bodies are where it's at!

For men, with the right exercises you can put on size, or if you're not into the body-builder look, you can create long, lean muscles, and washboard abs. But remember, even with the best-developed muscles, if you have a layer of fat covering them, you won't see those muscles. That's why the right combination of diet and exercise can transform your body and take years off of your looks. Seriously, it's amazing the things you can do through exercise.

In addition to weight lifting and strength training, cardio is great for your health and for weight loss. If you are going to add this type of workout regimen to your diet plan, it's important to consider what kind of exercise you enjoy. It's the same approach we have with food—if you don't like it, you're not going to stick with it. For example, I have a lot of respect for runners, but I don't run because I don't enjoy it. I'd rather go on the treadmill at a fast walking pace, or sign me up for a five-hour dance class any day! It's all relative.

You could go join a touch-football league or take a Hip-Hop class. Find a group of friends to go walking with, or join a hiking club. Whether it's running, tennis, soccer, martial arts, yoga, or dance, try and get involved in activities you like. When you do something you enjoy, it's more fun and effortless. Then you don't need to rely on willpower to push yourself to do it, and it is something you'll be more likely to stick with.

One of the nice things about realizing you don't need to work out in order to lose weight is that if you don't have time to work out, you don't need to worry. If you're too busy one day or can't make it to the gym, it won't be an excuse why you should go off your weight loss plan. Or if you are sick or need to take rest because of an injury, you don't have to wait until you are better to start trying to lose weight.

While adding an exercise regimen to your diet plan is not necessary, it will do wonders for your progress. In addition to burning extra calories, you'll notice that when you spend time working out, you'll be more motivated to stick to your weight loss plan. Plus, there is definitely a connection between clarity of mind and body. When you choose to keep your body healthy and in good shape, it will help your mind to stay sharp, clear, and focused. Overall, the better you take care of yourself, the better you will feel. And the better you feel, the easier it will be to achieve effortless weight loss.

CHAPTER 5

HAVE YOUR CAKE
AND EAT IT TOO

Life is really simple, but we insist on making it
complicated.

—Confucius

Over the years, people have come to believe that
weight loss is difficult, requires great sacrifice, and
means giving up your favorite food. Essentially, having
to choose between the body of your dreams and the food
you love. However, you don't need to choose between
the two because the two aren't mutually exclusive. You
see with calorie counting, you can essentially have your
cake and eat it too.

As an enlightened dieter, you will come to find that
not only can weight loss be easier, but it is entirely
possible to maintain your predilection for food and your
perfect weight. You see, like many things, successful
weight loss is similar to a lock and key. With the wrong
key you will find yourself flailing and struggling, but
with the right key, you can unlock your great potential
and achieve your perfect dream weight.

This chapter is dedicated to cleaning house when
it comes to some of the limiting beliefs you may be

carrying around concerning weight loss. Face it, whether it's from the media or past experiences—you may have negative feelings and attitudes when it comes to dieting and food. For example, do you think dieting is supposed to be difficult and grueling? Do you think it requires an indomitable willpower? Do you think weight-loss is hard and weight gain easy? What if I told you the opposite could be true. Or that it takes just as much energy to gain weight as it does to lose weight.

You see, whether you realize it or not, these very beliefs are affecting your success. So as part of your diet enlightenment work, I want you to forget everything you think you know about how difficult and challenging dieting is. Let go of the struggle and accept that weight loss can be perfectly natural. You see, with this philosophy, it's all about putting your attention on food in a certain way.

Let's start by discussing the word diet, which seems to elicit a knee jerk reaction from most people. The word has such a negative connotation that even some commerical weight loss companies have banned the word from their vocabulary—because apparently diets don't work, only lifestyle changes work. Well, we might be talking semantics here, but isn't it all the same thing? Whether you call it a diet, a weight loss plan, or a lifestyle change, it's about losing weight and keeping it off.

I don't think the problem lies in the concept of dieting; rather, it's that the majority of diets are painful, hard to stick to, and don't work long-term. But, what if you had a diet in which you were still eating the foods you enjoy, always feeling satisfied, and watching the weight fall of you? How could that be a bad thing? You see dieting doesn't need to have such a bad stigma.

This might sound strange, but when I think of the word diet, the only feelings that come to mind are ones of gratitude and appreciation. That's because I know I have a method that's easy to follow, easy to maintain, and works every time. Think back to other diets you tried that relied on willpower, and didn't it seem that the more you obsessed about losing weight the worse it seemed to go. That's because you were putting your attention on weight loss in the wrong way.

When you have a plan that makes you feel confident and at peace, you can develop a level of detachment and stop obsessing over it. Whether you attribute it to metaphysical laws or human psychology, there is no doubt that the way you think about things affects the outcome. It doesn't matter how many diets you've tried or how many years you've been at it because as an enlightened dieter now you're dieting efficiently. Trust me, you can feel great about weight loss because you know you are completely in control of your own destiny.

Let's take a moment to reflect on how truly lucky we are to live in a country in which we have access to unlimited food. It's a blessing that we often take for granted. Most of us don't have to worry about going hungry at night, eating whatever we can get our hands on, or wondering if we are even going to eat the next day. For many Americans, food is abundant and more convenient than ever. Ironically, our focus has shifted to whether or not we are skinny enough, and how we can avoid eating. I can't tell you how many people I've heard blame the convenience and availability of food on their weight problems.

Contrary to what you might think, I believe that having access to infinite food actually makes weight loss and maintenance easier, not harder. You see the more food and variety there is, the more freedom and options you have. You can scour the grocery stores for the perfect pasta that is both delicious and low-calorie. You can choose between five different brands of English muffins to find the one that is the best for you. You can look up the nutritional facts online before you go to a restaurant and choose your meals accordingly. Most importantly, you can stop eating when you are full because the food is still going to be there in the morning.

You see, while the rest of America is getting larger and blaming the food industry, I find it easier than ever to stay thin. Seriously, stop and be thankful that we live in a country in which food is abundant. Be thankful that we live in a time in which you can use the Internet to look up almost anything and find the nutritional facts. Be thankful that technology allows us to track our calories on the go, anytime, and anywhere. Despite what excuses you might hear, the truth is that in today's day and age, it is easier than ever to stay thin.

Another part of cleaning house involves not blaming your body and genetics. There seems to be this unspoken belief that if you're thin it's because you were blessed with perfect genes and if you're fat it's because you lost the genetic lottery. I'm sorry, but that doesn't make sense. The obesity rate in America has more than doubled since the 1980s, and it's because we are eating way too many calories—not because of genetic mutation. Genetics definitely have a role to play, but it's not what is making people overweight and obese—too many calories are.

I want to take a moment to address the physiological aspects of weight loss. While it is rare, I know that there are certain individuals who can eat as much as they want without gaining weight. Also, there are others who suffer from thyroid or metabolic conditions that contribute to weight gain and can make weight loss difficult. Now if you suspect that you are suffering from a medical issue that is interfering with your weight management, you should get checked out by a physician. However, I truly believe that for most of the population this is not a factor; it really is all about calorie consumption.

It's important to realize that for nearly all of us, it's not about family genetics or high and low metabolism; if you're overweight, it's probably because you are eating too many calories and not realizing it. Personally, I'm thin and it's not because of an awesome metabolism. It's because I maintain perfect weight control through calorie counting, portion control, and listening to my body. When I eat too many calories for an extended period of time, my weight goes up, and when I eat fewer calories, my weight goes down. It's as simple as that.

Look at Hollywood starlets such as Kristie Alley, Anna Nicole Smith, and Jessica Simpson. These ladies were the epitome of thin in their prime and you never would have guessed they would become overweight. However, despite being thin for most of their lives, they ended up seriously packing on the pounds. That's because if you consume too many calories for a long enough period of time, you will gain weight. On the other hand, look at celebrities such as Nicole Richie, Jennifer Hudson, and Randy Jackson—they did the exact opposite and lost the weight later in life, and have kept if off. Furthermore, look at Christina Aguilera, who was notoriously thin, then suddenly became heavy, and then lost the weight and became thin again.

So if the thin can become overweight and the overweight can become thin, then maybe there is more to it than genetics and metabolism. This is great news because it means you are in control of your own fate. It doesn't matter if you've been thin all of your life, if you suddenly start overeating and consuming way too many calories, you will gain weight. In contrast, there are lots of inspirational stories out there of individuals losing one or two hundred pounds, and thus achieving the so-called impossible. So whatever amount you have to lose, you should know that it is possible.

When it comes to cleaning house, you must discard some of the other limiting beliefs and stereotypes about "fat people". For example, there seems to be this pervasive belief in our society that overweight people lack self-control and discipline. So does it just happen to be that all the heavy people lack will power, and all the skinny people have amazing will power? No, that doesn't seem right, and it's not true.

After all, I know thin people that lack self-control with their finances, substance abuse, etc. On the other hand, I know heavier people who struggle with their weight, but demonstrate amazing self-control and determination in other areas of their life. Plus, isn't the person who tries diet after diet, year after year, despite failure after failure demonstrating perseverance and fortitude? There has to be something else at work here.

I thought back to my own experiences in the past and realized that the times I needed to rely on willpower to stick to a diet, I just didn't have much success. Yet, when I finally did take the weight off for good, it kind of felt effortless. Why was that? It wasn't because I dug deep and reached a new level of self-discipline. Rather, it was because I changed my thinking and approach, and it became easier. Now don't get me wrong, successful calorie counting requires creativity, enthusiasm, planning, consistency, and great attention-to-detail; but it just doesn't require half the will-power of most other diets.

Many of us who've failed at dieting in the past, assume it's physiological or that we just lack the determination to succeed. Society sure leads us to believe this. While it's perfectly understandable why you might feel this way, it's more likely that your dieting program lacks substance and not you. I'm telling you there is a key to making weight loss easier, and making it stick for the long-term. Also, I'm going to let you in on a little secret about most thin people. But before we get to that I want to tell you about my younger sisters.

Everyone in my family jokes that my youngest sister on my mom's side can eat anything she wants without ever gaining weight. Most people shrug it off that she's still growing or has a super fast metabolism. Granted she's thirteen years younger, but I think there is more to it. Obviously, she never worries about gaining or losing weight, she eats constantly throughout the day, and orders whatever she wants. But here is the kicker—she never ends up eating that much because she gets full.

Seriously, my husband and I will take her out for dinner, and she'll order the most fattening thing on the menu, but barely eats half of it. Then two hours later we take her out for Ice cream, she orders the small size and doesn't even finish it. Three hours later she's hungry again, asks for a sandwich and has two bites. She eats whatever she wants, whenever she's hungry, but she always stops when she's satisfied. At the end of the day, she just doesn't end up consuming that many calories.

I have another younger sister on my dad's side who does the same thing. She's always been thin and eats whatever she wants, but she doesn't actually eat that much. I've even witnessed her stop eating with only a few bites left. Seriously what teenager gets a bag of Cheetos and doesn't finish them all! I remember asking her "Why did you stop and not finish it?" Her answer was so simple and yet profound. She said, "Why would I continue eating when I'm full? I can always finish it later." She was right; it seems thin people just don't feel the need to overeat.

I started to notice a pattern; not just with my younger sisters, but also with certain adults. For example, I went out to dinner with an older friend of mine who was always very slim. On this particular night, I remember she ordered the Fettuccini Alfredo, but only ate half. It's not like she portioned it out, but rather she took her time eating as we talked, and she stopped when she was full. Then half an hour later, she ordered the Brownie Delight for dessert, had a few bites, and brought the rest home for her husband. The truth was, despite ordering two of the most fattening things on the menu, she really didn't end up eating that many calories.

This whole thing got me thinking about all of the skinny people out there who appear to eat whatever they want. If only a small percentage of people actually suffer from metabolic disorders, then why were all these thin people eating whatever they wanted and staying thin. What I realized was that it's really more of an illusion that most thin people can eat whatever they want without gaining weight. In reality, they don't end up eating that many calories or as many calories as you'd think. You see—when you have a healthy relationship with food and listen to your body, you naturally eat the right portions and stay thin.

If you start paying attention to the behavior of those who've have been thin all of their life, you'll notice something interesting. While they may seem to eat whatever they want and whenever they want, they always stop when they are full and they don't overeat or binge. I noticed this behavior with my mom and my step-mom, both of whom had always been thin. I started noticing it with certain cousins, friends, and coworkers. I even started seeing it in the behavior and in the dialogue of strangers at restaurants. It seemed that thin people operated from an entirely different mind-set than those struggling with their weight.

It appears that the naturally thin person operates from an abundance mentality. With the example of my older friend, she eats whatever she wants, she stops when she's satisfied, and doesn't give it another thought. She feels good, her thoughts are positive, and she doesn't worry about food or her weight. Because of this abundance mentality, food doesn't represent that siren call that it does for many others.

The typical dieter on the other hand, operates from a scarcity mentality. I don't mean scarcity in that they think they might wake up and not have food tomorrow. Rather, I mean scarcity in that they limit the food they think they can eat and make certain foods off-limits. Also, they believe that dieting is extremely difficult and that they need to be perfect to achieve their goal. It's really this scarcity mentality that makes dieters stressed about weight loss and causes them to sabotage their own efforts.

So the next time you go out to dinner, pay attention to the eating behaviors of different types of people. The naturally thin person who is maintaining their weight will probably have one dinner roll, a few bites of an appetizer, and then wait for their entrée. They'll eat slowly, savor the food, and they won't stress about eating. Because they are thin and it takes less to make them feel full, they'll stop when they are satisfied and probably only end up eating two-thirds or half of their entrée, especially if it's a very large portion.

On the other hand, your typical dieter will try their best not to have any bread, but then if they give in, they'll end up eating the whole basket. They'll feel bad, polish off their entrée—which is probably a deceptive high calorie salad—and possibly eat some of yours. Then as some sort of self-sabotaging punishment, they'll order the most fattening thing on the dessert menu and eat all of it. And yes, they'll declare they are starting their diet again on Monday!

See for your serial dieter, it's always black and white. You're either being perfect or you're off your diet, and when you're off your diet that's a license to binge. The typical dieter's mentality is that when they are good they are great, but when they have a moment of weakness and eat something they think they are not supposed to, they rationalize by going off the deep-end. It's that type of thinking that leads to unhealthy relationships with food.

I've noticed that when you obsess about food and weight loss, you end up manifesting the same situation over and over again. If you focus too much on needing to lose weight and how difficult it is, your experience will be exactly that. You start to drive yourself crazy and sabotage your own efforts. However, when you have faith and a rock-solid plan, you can develop some level of detachment from the situation, and things start to change quickly. It's not a coincidence. Your mental attitude and emotions have a huge impact on your ability to lose weight.

When done correctly, losing weight and maintaining it should not be a struggle. Weight loss is not all or nothing and one "bad" meal can never sabotage your efforts unless you allow it to. That's why if you can change the way you see dieting, you can change your experience. As you become an enlightened dieter, you'll learn how to think and behave like a naturally thin person. Down the road, you might even be mistaken for one of those "lucky ones" with an awesome metabolism.

Another interesting factor to consider is that your stomach is flexible and adaptive. If you continue to overeat, you will gain weight, stretch your stomach out, and it will take more food to make you feel full. By the same token, the thinner you are, the smaller your stomach is, and the less food you need to feel full. When you are thin, it's easier to stay thin because you get full quicker. More importantly, when you learn how to listen to your body and have a healthy relationship with food, it actually becomes more difficult to gain weight.

I want you to use your imagination for a second and envision that I am sitting down for dinner at a pizza parlor with another woman. In this example, we're both 5'2", but I weigh 105 pounds and the other woman weighs 300 pounds. Now if we were both instructed to eat slices of pizza until we were completely satisfied, the amount of food we would both need to eat would be significantly different. The other woman might need to eat 8-10 slices, while I would feel totally satisifed after 2-3 slices. And guess what? We would both be reaching the same level of fullness.

Do you grasp the gravity of what I'm getting at here? When you are thin, it takes much less food to make you full. So you get to enjoy that same euphoric satisfied feeling as the woman sitting across from you—the difference is, I'm going to remain thin and she's going to remain overweight. A few slices of pizza are well within my calorie budget for dinner , but 8-10 slices in one meal would make anyone gain weight.

If you think about it, there is no downside to losing weight and becoming thinner. You see when you're thin, it's easier to stay thin because it takes so much less to make you full, and you still get to enjoy food. I've noticed the real difference between naturally thin people and those struggling to lose weight is the way they think about food. If you want to make sure you stay thin, then you must change the way you relate to food. Change your thoughts and you'll change your life.

So unless you've been diagnosed with an actual medical disorder, stop blaming family genetics or your metabolism. Even if you do have a syndrome that makes weight loss difficult, the techniques in this book can still help you lose weight. I've seen people with medical issues defy science and achieve what they knew in their hearts they could accomplish. Sometimes the greatest roadblocks and limitations are the ones in our minds. So the next time someone tells you that you can't have your cake and eat it too, you know that you can—you just have to count your calories.

CHAPTER 6
THE ART OF CALORIE COUNTING

See first that the design is wise and just; that
ascertained, pursue it resolutely.

—William Shakespeare

I once heard someone declare that counting calories
is no way to live! Well I say that being overweight,
not having the body of your dreams, and not eating
the food you love is no way to live! Bottom line—if
you want to lose weight, you need to monitor what
you eat in one way or another. This is true whether
you're eliminating specific food, limiting your portions,
following a set plan of meals, counting your points,
or counting your calories. And while there are many
approaches to weight loss, I find calorie counting by far
the simplest and easiest method. You can't argue with
science—eat more calories than you burn and you will
gain weight; eat fewer calories than you burn and you
will lose weight.

Despite the fact that calorie counting is a proven
method to lose weight and keep it off, many people
still reach for the latest fad diets. It always baffles me
when I meet individuals who have given up on weight
loss, yet they haven't even given calorie counting a

chance. Some people shy away from the whole "calorie counting" thing because they assume it will be tedious and annoying, but in reality it's incredibly easy, strangely rewarding, and works marvelously.

What I especially like about calorie counting is that it can accommodate any eating style. Whether you are a vegetarian, a diabetic, a health-nut, or a carb-lover like me, it gives you the freedom to choose food based on your prerogative. Calorie counting can work for anyone because it's flexible and fits individuals' tastes and preferences. In fact, it's impossible for it not to work as long as it is done correctly. Trust me—counting your calories is a small price to pay for staying thin and getting to eat whatever you want.

When it comes to dieting, doesn't it seem like the next new diet always claims to be revolutionary? Well I'm here to tell you that there is nothing new or revolutionary about calorie counting. In fact, it's one of the oldest dieting methods around. You may be thinking to yourself, if it's been around this long, why do so many people struggle with weight loss today?

Well, before the low-carbohydrate diets became all the rage, dietary advice was simple—consume fewer calories than you burn and you will lose weight. But today, dieting is all about counting your carbs, reducing your fats, and other diet trends and gimmicks. It's no surprise that diets are failing, and Americans aren't getting any thinner.

Another interesting factor to consider is that just because people have heard of calorie counting doesn't mean that they know how to do it correctly. Believe it or not, there are a few different schools of thought or formulas when it comes to calorie counting. But don't worry; by the end of this chapter, you'll have great confidence and know exactly what you need to do in order to lose weight. Trust me; there is an art to calorie counting that makes it simple and work every time.

The secret to mastering weight loss can really be broken up into three main concepts. The first part is the art of calorie counting; that is the scientific formula for determining how many calories you need to lose weight. The second part is the art of choosing what you eat; which is how you will spend your calories, and is the key to sticking to your plan and making it effortless. The third part is the art of listening to your body; which is essentially, learning when to eat and how to eat for the right reasons.

This dieting philosophy will work flawlessly when all three parts of the formula are applied. But don't worry because these three parts go together like graham crackers, marshmallows, and chocolate. Remember, successful weight loss is not achieved through struggle; it's achieved through ease and peace of mind. We'll get to part two and three in later chapters, but for now, let's explore—what is a calorie, how does calorie counting work, and what is this age-old formula for weight loss success.

So what exactly is a calorie? According to Merriam-Webster dictionary, a calorie is defined as a unit equivalent to the large calorie expressing heat-producing or energy-producing value in food when oxidized in the body; or an amount of food having an energy-producing value of one large calorie.[16] In laymen's terms, calories are the energy in food. And, regardless of where they come from—carbohydrate, protein, or fat—they're either burned up or stored within your body.

I'm not going to bore you with the science behind calories and weight loss. The neat thing about calories is that you don't need to be a scientist or nutritionist to understand how to count them. It's like when you learn how to drive a car, you don't need to know the mechanics of the engine or the physics behind why the car works; you just learn how to drive and you get where you need to go. So, let's learn how to drive.

1. DETERMINE YOUR DAILY CALORIE NEEDS

The first step to losing weight is to figure out your daily calorie needs—that is the total number of calories you need to maintain your current weight. Throughout this book I will also refer to this number as your maintenance number. If you were to consume this amount of calories each day you would neither gain nor lose weight. We always start with this number and then work our way backwards.

If you type in "Daily Calorie Needs" in any search engine, you'll find plenty of websites with free online calculators that will help you figure out your daily calorie requirements. If you spend enough time searching for these types of calculators you'll notice that they don't all necessarily give you the same number. That's because not all online calculators are created equal; some use different formulas such as Mifflin-St Joer, Katch-McCardle, or Harris-Benedict.

In 2005, the American Dietetic Association (ADA) published a comparison of the various equations and found the Mifflin-St Joer formula to be the most accurate. Also, according to Nutrition Therapy and Pathophysiology, the Mifflin-St. Joer equation has been validated by more than ten studies.[17] I've also personally experimented with all three formulas and found Mifflin-St Joer to be the most effective.

While you'll find that some popular calculators still use the Harris-Benedict equation, the Mifflin-St. Jeor equation is the most reliable formula, and it's the one that we'll be using in this book. There is no reason to worry about which calculators use which formulas because I'll show you the best free online calculator to use based on this equation.

It's important to recognize that any daily calorie needs calculator will only give you an estimated number. Given that muscle mass, fat distribution, and metabolic rate vary from person to person, actual calories needed to maintain weight can fluctuate slightly. Nevertheless, this estimated number is extremely effective, and can be used to achieve incredible results with weight loss. This is the formula that I personally have used, as well as all of my clients, to lose the weight and keep it off for good.

The best online Daily Calorie Needs calculator that is free, easy to use, and based on the Mifflin St. Joer equation is available on the website FreeDieting.com. The below URL will take you to the Calculator page where you can determine the amount of daily calories you need to maintain your current weight—also known as maintenance. You can also find a link to this calculator on my website listed below.

www.freedieting.com/calorie-calculator

www.dietenlightenment.com/links

The above online calculator takes into consideration your gender, age, current weight, height, and activity/exercise level. Believe it or not, the older you are, the fewer calories you need to maintain your weight. Did you know that you get way more calories just for being a guy—I know it's not fair! As for height, it makes a huge difference in relation to your weight. Think about it, 130 pounds on a woman five feet tall will look completely different than on a woman who is 5'8" tall. Also, the less you weigh, the less calories you need to maintain your weight. Remember, the daily calorie needs number is the number you need to maintain your current weight—we'll get to calculating the losing weight part in a second.

If you are interested, you can look up the complete Mifflin-St. Joer equation online and do it by hand. However, unless you are a math fanatic, I definitely recommend you use the simple online calculator to save you time and avoid human error. Now this is important—while the first four fields on the daily needs calculator are pretty straight forward, I have an important suggestion when it comes to the activity/ exercise category that I believe will make your calculation much more accurate. I recommend that you do not account for exercise when determining your daily calorie needs, but instead add in your exercise calories later. This way, you know what your maintenance number is, regardless of whether you exercise or not on a certain day. In a minute, I'll show you how to account for your exercise calories in the best way possible.

Think about it—it doesn't make sense to generalize exercise calories for everyone. For example, if three different people were to select "exercise moderately 3-5 days per week" it could mean three very different scenarios. Keep in mind that not all exercise is created equal when it comes to burning calories, and different people burn different amounts of calories for the same activity.

Plus, what one person considers moderate might mean something completely different to the next person. I find it much more scientific to figure out how many calories you burned for a specific workout and then add it to your daily calories. Therefore, when it comes to the activity/exercise field, you should really be asking yourself what you do during the day. Do you have a desk job or similar activity level? Are you doing hard physical labor for work? Or are you an athlete intensely working out more than five hours a day, more than five days a week.

Now if you are a professional athlete, you should select the higher activity level. However, if you are like most people and have a regular job, I recommend you select the sedentary or little/no exercise option. It doesn't matter if you workout every single night, you can still select the little/no exercise option because you are going to add in your exercise calories later. You see, you're still accounting for all your exercise; you're just doing it much more precisely.

Another reason I like this approach is because it offers more flexibility. People get sick, have to stay late at work, or something comes up that interferes with working out. If for some reason you don't get to exercise, your daily calorie needs won't be affected.

Personally, I can't always guarantee how often I'm going to exercise until I actually do it. Some weeks it's like Jillian Michaels and other weeks it's more like Homer Simpson. I like having the flexibility to know my daily calorie needs with or without exercise. When I do exercise, I just add those additional calories that day. The choice is up to you, but the more accurate you are, the better results you will get.

To help demonstrate the daily calorie needs calculation, let's use a fictitious person. Let's say this individual is female, 30 years old, 5'6" and weighs 150 pounds. If you use the above calculator and select the little/no exercise option, you'll see her maintenance number is roughly 1,700 calories per day. If she were to consume this amount of calories every day, her weight would stay the same.

Now use the online calculator to determine your daily calorie needs, and then we'll figure out how many fewer calories you need to lose weight.

2. DETERMINE HOW MANY CALORIES YOU NEED TO LOSE WEIGHT

Once you know your daily calorie needs for your current weight, which is your maintenance number, then you can figure out how many fewer calories you need to lose weight. It's simple—you take your maintenance number and subtract 20 percent.

For example , if your maintenance number is 1,700 calories then 20 percent of that is 340 calories. 1,700 calories minus 340 calories equals 1,360 calories. So your magic weight loss number would be 1,360 calories per day! And, as you lose weight, you would need to recalculate your daily calorie needs and apply the 20 percent rule. That's pretty much how this works in a nutshell.

Before you run upstairs to get your TI-83 calculator, you'll notice that the online calculator I gave you automatically does both calculations for you— your maintenance number and your fat loss number. Ignore the extreme fat loss number, and only pay attention to the maintenance and fat loss. I'll explain why later!

Theoretically, you can achieve the 20 percent deficit by eating fewer calories, burning more calories, or a combination of both. However, as we discussed in Chapter 4, it is unlikely that exercise alone will compensate for this difference. While working out can definitely help you burn some additional calories, I recommend that you put your focus and attention on what you consume.

Many experts recommend that calories should never dip below 1,200 for women and 1,700 for men However, I think it's difficult to establish one set of minimum calorie requirements for everyone. Does it make sense that a woman six-feet tall with a large frame should have the same minimum calorie requirements as a woman 4'10" with a small frame? I don't think so! You'd also be surprised to find that someone with the exact same height and weight as you but many years older or younger may require very different calories. Nonetheless, I still agree with guidelines because it's important to have minimum calorie requirements, since having too little calories is bad for your health and for your diet.

For many people, the above calculation will never put you below 1,200 calories for women and 1,700 calories for men. However, in some cases, if you are petite or older, you might notice that it does. And that's okay. It's important to note that the smaller you are, the fewer calories you require. Also, as you get older, you require fewer calories too. Keep in mind, that this number still hasn't even accounted for your additional exercise calories yet in case you are really active.

So in these specific cases, I think it is okay to amend the minimum weight loss calorie requirements to 1,100 for women and 1,600 for men. I know it might not seem like much of a difference, but this is the absolute lowest you should ever go. Now this doesn't mean you should consume 1,100 calories if your calculation says 1,180. What it means is even if the calculation puts you below 1,100 for women or 1,600 for men, you should always stay above that number no matter what.

Plus, as I said before, you can add additional calories for exercise. We want fat loss, not extreme fat loss, which is why these minimum calorie requirements are important to follow. Trust me; there is no reason to ever go under these calorie requirements. Not only is it bad for your health, but also you don't need to in order to lose weight effectively.

I've tried the extreme 800 and 1,000-calorie diets in the past; not only was it difficult, but also it just didn't work that well. Besides water weight, you don't actually lose any real weight faster. When it comes to the Mifflin St. Joer formula and the 20 percent rule, there really seems to be magic in this equation. So stick to your weight loss number, and don't go lower than these guidelines.

If for some reason you decide that you don't want to go below 1,200 calories for women and 1,700 calories for men, that's fine. You will still lose weight, it'll just be significantly slower. For instance, you may choose to be conservative and consume 15 percent fewer calories instead of 20 percent. Again, the great thing about this diet is that you can customize it to work for you.

However, if you are trying to lose weight as efficiently as possible while still staying healthy, 20 percent is your magic number.

When you follow the 20 percent rule, you'll typically lose between 1-3 pounds per week. If you're working on those last five pounds, keep in mind that 0.5 to 1 pound per week is a safe and reasonable rate. However if you have a lot to lose, you might find yourself losing more weight even faster. Because humans aren't robots there is no guaranteed number for how much weight you will lose per week; some weeks you'll lose a little more and some weeks a little less. But if you stick to these guidelines, you will eventually lose all the weight you want guaranteed.

Use the above calculator and the 20 percent rule to determine your weight loss number—how many calories you should consume each day to lose weight. Remember that as you lose weight, your body will require fewer calories and you should update your daily calorie requirements for weight loss accordingly.

3. HOW TO ADD IN EXERCISE CALORIES

As long as you properly account for your calories burned through exercise, you can apply them to your daily calorie goal with great results. For example, let's say your weight loss number is 1,200 calories; if you eat 1,200 calories and complete an 80 calorie workout, you can confidently eat an additional 80 calories that day and still be at 1,200 calories. Make sense?

Incorporating exercise can be a great tool to burn extra calories and help you stick to your weight loss number. Keep in mind, I'm talking about exercise calories here, and not general activity calories . If you wanted to, you could actually calculate how many calories you burned for doing the laundry, making dinner, or even getting up to go to the printer. But, we have already accounted for these basic daily calories in our daily calorie needs equation.

What I'm talking about here is actual moderate to hardcore exercise. For example, walking steeply uphill on the treadmill, going for a run, playing an intense basketball game, taking a spinning class, etc. These are the types of exercise calories that you can add to your weight loss number. You can even think about exercise calories like coupons. For example, if you ate 1,400 calories, but then did an intense one hundred calorie workout, it's like having a coupon for one hundred calories off! It's a funny way of looking at it, but it's true.

It's important to recognize that most people significantly overestimate the calories they burn through exercise. I can't emphasize this enough! You can't always rely on your treadmill or elliptical machine to tell you how many calories you burned. For example, when I go on the treadmill for thirty minutes at 3.5 mph it says I burned 260 calories. That is probably correct for a 185 pound male. However since I'm only 5'2" and 105 pounds, that's pretty unlikely. In reality, I know I only burned roughly one hundred calories.

So then the question becomes—how do you most accurately determine how many calories you burned through exercise? It's easy! You can use an online activity "calories burned" calculator that takes into consideration your gender, age, height, weight, and duration and intensity of the activity. It is similar to the calculator we use to figure out your daily calorie needs.

Bear in mind, that any activity calculator can only provide you with an estimate. However, since it's based on your individual factors, it's very reliable. I find that this approach is much more accurate than using a universal number made for everyone that doesn't take into consideration your size.

My favorite free resource for determining calories burned is the "calories burned exercise calculator" available at:

www.freedieting.com/calories-burned

This calculator uses the latest figures from the Compendium of Physical Activities, which is a publication from Arizona State University.[19] Whatever online calculator you choose, just make sure it takes into consideration your gender, age, height, and weight.

When it comes to this calculation, you have to be as accurate as possible. My recommendation is that if you are not sure how many exercise calories you burned, it's always better to underestimate. As you start using these exercise/activity calculators, you'll get more confident with adding back in your exercise calories to your overall number.

The great thing about this approach is that if you set out to do a light workout, but end up doing an intense workout or vice versa, you can just adjust your calories accordingly. Or, if you go over your daily calorie goal, you can jump on the treadmill and burn off those extra calories. Lastly, if you aren't able to work out on a specific day, don't worry because you already know your daily calorie goal without exercise. Having this type of flexibility when it comes to working out and losing weight will help you stay on track long-term.

I'm often asked whether or not you absolutely need to add back in your exercise calories. That is a personal choice. You can choose to skip adding back in your exercise calories for more extreme weight loss. However, I personally like to add back in my exercise calories because I believe it provides a more accurate number. It is my experience, as well as many of my clients, that as long as you don't overestimate your exercise calories when adding them back in, you will have the best results. So use your best judgement. For example, if you do a light twenty minute workout, it is understandable to not add back in those calories. However, if you decide to do a super intense workout such as training for a marathon, taking a spinning class, or going hiking up hill, then I would recommend adding back in those calories.

4. STAY WITHIN YOUR CALORIE RANGE

Once you know your weight loss number, you should always strive to consume as close to this number as possible. The more consistently you do this, the more quickly and efficiently you will lose weight. For example, if your weight loss number is 1,280 and your maintenance number is 1,600, try to stick to 1,280 calories per day. However, since we can't always be perfect, it's important to know that as long as you consume somewhere between your weight loss number and your maintenance number, you won't hinder your weight loss.

Think about it—if your maintenance number keeps you at the same weight and your weight loss number helps you lose weight, then staying in between the two numbers is kind of like a safety net. Again, always strive to hit the weight loss target number, but if you happen to go over, just stay within your range and don't give it another thought.

Having a range also gives you flexibility for times when you may need to use extra calories. In fact, something that I used to do was Monday through Friday, I'd eat my exact weight loss number or close to it. Then on Saturday and Sunday, I would throw myself an extra few hundred calories if needed. Also if I knew I had a special dinner coming up, I would stick to my weight loss number all week and then possibly use those extra calories for that dinner.

You may find that you never want or need to go above your weight loss number calories. In fact, if you never use them, you will lose weight as quickly and efficiently as possible. However, it's nice to know that you have a safety net, and as long as you stay within your calorie range you will still lose weight.

Think about weight loss in terms of a large staircase. If you perpetually take five steps down and then march in place, and then take another five steps down and march in place again, you've still moving down the staircase, and will eventually get to the bottom. It's like that with weight loss. The better you stick to your weight loss number, the faster you'll go down, but even if you go down slowly, you'll still get there.

Now if you're walking down the staircase and accidently go a step or two in the wrong direction, just pick up where you left off. Don't throw yourself down the staircase or run back up and start over. That's loco! Unfortunately, that's exactly what a lot of dieters do; they take a few steps in the wrong direction and assume they blew it. Then they go on a weekend-long caloric binge and undo all the progress they made that week.

That's as silly as throwing yourself down the stairs or running back up to start over. So if you go over your weight loss number, you can either burn the extra calories through exercise or just stay within your range. When it comes to losing weight, it's not all or nothing. You don't need to be perfect all of the time to lose weight. Even if worst comes to worst you happen to go above your range, no worries—one bad meal or day can never unravel weeks of progress. Regardless of a blip here and there, it won't make a difference as long as you keep the course.

Remember, if you want to lose weight as efficiently as possible, always stick to your weight loss number or as close to it as possible. As you learn to master the art of what you eat, you'll find it easier to stick to this number. However, it's still nice to know that you always have your safety net to catch you.

QUICK SUMMARY

Use the daily caloric needs calculator listed below (based on the Mifflin-St Joer Formula) to determine how many calories you need each day in order to maintain your current weight; this is your maintenance number. It is recommended that you do not account for exercise as part of this equation, but rather add in exercise calories separately based on individual workouts.

Take your maintenance number and subtract 20 percent to figure out how many calories you need each day to lose weight; this is your weight loss number and your daily target goal. If you need to consume additional calories, just make sure you stick between your weight loss number and maintenance number.

The cool thing about the below online calculator is that it determines both your maintenance number and weight loss number at the same time. I've also listed below the calories burned calculator so you can determine roughly how many calories you burn for a specific workout. You can then add back in these exercise calories to help you reach your daily calorie goal or stay within your budget.

Quick Links:

www.freedieting.com/calorie-calculator

www.freedieting.com/calories-burned

CHAPTER 7

KEEPING TRACK OF YOUR CALORIES

He who fails to plan, plans to fail.

—Sir Winston Churchill

Keeping track of your calories is very much like keeping a budget. When you have a budget, you keep track of how much money you have and know how much money you can spend. It's as simple as that. Before the days of credit cards, we were all a lot better at this. But even credit cards have maximum limits; and if you use credit cards, you have to pay them off each month unless you want to pay interest. Budgeting your calories is no different! In fact, it's something you already do in many areas of your life.

For example, let's say you left your credit cards at home, and go to the mall with $200 cash. You know how much money you can spend and can see how much different items cost. You'll then make decisions based on what you want and how much money you have. Do you want to spend all of your cash on a $200 shirt or buy ten shirts at a less expensive store? Or, let's say you've already spent most of your money and then find a nice pair of pants, but you don't have enough money left over. You'll either come back tomorrow with more money or you'll find something similar that's within your budget.

If shopping isn't your thing you can also think about it in terms of budgeting for your household. We all have different types of expenses that we have to manage each month. Even if you plan on using credit cards to help cover your expenses, if you're going to stay within your budget and not go into debt, you still need to pay off your credit cards and cover your bills each month. Budgeting is an important skill that you already use whether it's at home, at work, or even just out on a shopping trip.

And, just like if you continuously go over your financial budget, you'll eventually go into debt. If you do the same thing with your calories, you'll end up gaining weight. On the other hand, losing weight is simple because all you need to do is stay within your calorie budget. Even if you're new to budgeting, keeping track of your calories can be easy. All you have to do is know how many calories you want to consume each day, keep track of what you eat, and make sure you stay within your budget. It doesn't matter if you've never been good at math or finance, you can still be great at calorie counting.

Think of your daily calorie needs to lose weight— also known as your weight loss number—as the cash in your wallet. It's the money you have to work with each day. For example, if you have $100 in your wallet and have a $60 haircut that afternoon including tip, then you know you can only spend an additional $40 that day.

The same goes for your calories. If you have 1,400 calories per day and you know you're going out to the Cheesecake Factory that night and want to order the 600-calorie Skinnylicious Shrimp Tacos, then you know you have 800 calories to use the rest of the day.

If your weight loss number is the proverbial cash in your wallet, then the additional calories in your range, up to your maintenance number, would be your "mad money." For those of you who aren't familiar with the concept of "mad money," it's something from my parents' generation. When people used to go out, they'd put some extra cash away in a hiding spot for emergencies. That's how your additional calories should work. Plan on not using them, but if you need to, they're there as a safety net.

And yes, just as you'll still be within your budget if you occasionally use your "mad money," you will still lose weight even when you use your extra calories now and then. The more you use your "mad money" or additional calories, the slower your weight loss will be; however, you will still lose weight. While most days you should have no problem sticking to your weight loss number, it's nice to know you have those extra calories if you need them.

I will warn you that during your first few weeks of counting your calories it will likely be an eye-opening experience. Most people don't realize how many calories are actually in the food they eat. This is especially true when it comes to some of the so-called diet or health foods that surprisingly pack a lot of calories. If you had trouble losing weight with other diets, or didn't lose weight despite just eating healthier, paying attention to your calories will help you understand where you may have went wrong in the past.

Unlike other popular diets, what makes the diet enlightenment approach so simple is that there is no need to document carbs, fats, sugar, or protein; the only thing you are tracking is your calories. If you also want to keep an eye on these things for health reasons that's fine, but it's not part of this program or even necessary to lose weight. Remember, as an enlightened dieter you eat healthy for your health, but eat the right amount of calories for your waistline.

In the previous chapter, you figured out your weight loss number and maintenance number. Since you already know your calorie budget, now it's time to decide how you're going to keep track of your calories. You could use a notebook, a word document, or even an excel spreadsheet, but it is the 21st century! The best and absolute easiest way to track your calories is to use an online calorie tracker because all of the calculations are done for you.

There are lots of free, online tools that can help you record what you eat and track your calories. Plus, most of these programs have extensive food libraries or databases to help you figure out the different calories in food. Whether you use a calorie tracker website or an iPhone app, these resources are amazing tools that make calorie counting incredibly easy and convenient.

Here is a list of free online calorie trackers that I'd recommend. I also list these URLS on my personal website, and I keep it updated as I find new ones.

1. www.livestrong.com/myplate

2. www.myfitnesspal.com

3. www.fatsecret.com

4. www.mynetdiary.com

5. www.sparkpeople.com

Personally, I like to use the Livestrong MyPlate calorie tracker. Their website, which syncs up with their iPhone app, allows you to track your caloric intake for all your meals and has an option to log your workout calories. Not only does it have a good user-experience for tracking what you eat, it also has a great database for looking up the calories in various foods. And, if you can't find what you are looking for, just search the Internet and add it manually.

Now this is important! As differenct apps/websites use different formulas for caloric needs, make sure to avoid using their preset daily calorie needs number. We've already determined your weight loss number and maintenance number, and you can add your calorie goals to the program manually. And remember, as you lose weight, update your weight loss number and adjust your budget accordingly. All you need to do is enter the food you eat, select the quantity, and the program automaticallys adds up the calories for you.

I even use this application to plan out my meals ahead of time. And, if what I eat changes, I just update it in the system and adjust the calories for the rest of the day accordingly. Whichever method you choose for tracking your calories, make sure it's something that's helpful and easily accessible.

I can't stress enough how important it is to record what you eat every day. Even if you are not proud of what you ate, you still need to record it regardless. Logging your food intake each day will start to make you more mindful of what you eat and your eating habits. Research has shown that people who keep a daily food journal or record what they eat, are likely to lose twice as much weight as those who don't.

For those of you who've never counted calories before, you might be a little concerned that this could be difficult or time-consuming. Just like any new habit, it will take some time getting used to, but it's actually quite simple. Once you get the hang of it, you'll realize how easy it is. It'll be like logging on to Facebook every day. The difference is you'll probably spend way more time on Facebook. Plus, the more you track your calories, the better and faster you'll get at it. It's really nothing more than a few clicks after every meal and then you're done.

In fact, it's never been easier to look up calories. Twenty years ago, you had a physical calorie book that you had to carry around with you. And if a particular item wasn't in there, then you didn't know the calories and had to guess. These days, you can find the calories for practically anything online. Even for something as obscure as Hungarian Goulash.

Remember, you're looking up calories ahead of time, so you can design delicious meals that will keep you feeling full and happy. Choose your meals like an artist chooses their color palette. It shouldn't feel like work . Rather , be creative with it and have fun. The people that have the most success with this find themselves actually enjoying planning their meals out ahead of time —almost like a game . While you are spending time thinking about what you want to eat, you're not really thinking about losing weight; rather you're coming up with exciting meals to help you feel great throughout the day.

I think it's helpful if you think of checking calories like checking the price tag in a store. You wouldn't go to the mall and purchase things without checking the price? So why would you eat things without checking the calories? If you're not careful, you could end up with a $5,000 purse or a five-hundred calorie muffin. You want to make sure your budget can afford it before you get it. Plus , it's not uncommon to have to ask the sales-clerk for a price check or scan the item to find out the price. Looking up your calories isn't that big of a stretch.

There are a few different ways to figure out the calories in food. When it comes to packaged food, all you have to do is look at the label for the nutritional facts. Most packaged foods have the nutritional facts on the back, which include the calories. When it comes to packaging, make sure you check the serving size. Some food companies are clever and make the calories low, but reduce the serving size. Whether you're picking something up from the grocery store or grabbing something from the cafeteria, just check the back for the calories to see what you're working with.

Now for foods that don't have packaging that lists the calories, all you need to do is look it up online or in your calorie tracker database. With the Internet and smart phones, it's easy and convenient to look up calories For example, go to Google search engine and type in Calories McDonald's Hamburger. Ta-duh! Within one click, you'll have your answer. Or you could have gone directly to the McDonald's website nutrition facts page to look upthe calories. Now I'm not at all suggesting McDonald's hamburgers here, but trying to illustate a point. There are so many resources available to figure out the calories in different foods.

Thanks to the fact that certain cities now require restaurant chains to make their nutritional facts available, you can look up almost any chain restaurant and get the nutritional information online. As time goes on, more and more restaurants will provide their nutritional information, or offer tools that make calorie counting even easier.

Even if you're going to a restaurant that doesn't list its nutritional information online, you can still look up the menu ahead of time and figure out the calorie approximations for different meals with a little research. In chapter 10 of this book, I will explain a technique for when you're going to someone's house or out to a restaurant and can't look it up ahead of time. These days, most restaurants have their menus online, so you can check it out before you go there.

There are many free tools to help you figure out the calories in food. You can use the database in your calorie tracker, check the restaurant's website, or research it on the Internet. Here are a few free resources that can also help you look up calories:

1. www.nutritionix.com
2. www.calorieking.com
3. http://calorielab.com

Nutritionix is one of my favorite websites for researching calories. In addition to its food database, it has a nutrition calculator that allows you to customize orders at your favorite restaurants, and it automatically tallies up the calories for you. For example, go to the Nutritionix Subway Nutrition Calculator and build your sandwich from scratch. It's especially great for someone like me who's always personalizing orders.

When it comes to preparing dinner at home, it's the same approach. All you need to do is tally up the calories in the individual ingredients and add it to your calorie tracker. For example, if you're making a sandwich and it's two slices of breads, five slices of turkey, one slice of cheese, and two tablespoons of mustard—just add up the calories for all of the different items.

Also, when it comes to eating at home, I would definitely invest in a food scale, and measuring cups and spoons. Soon enough you'll be able to eyeball portions. For example, I know exactly how much cream cheese to put on my English muffin to equal two tablespoons.

Plus, this will help you when you're not at home and are unable to measure. Your brain will start to become very good at portion sizes. You can even use your hand, or a spoon to help you gauge portions.

Another important key to tracking your calories is to be as accurate as possible with your portions. For example, if it says one cup of Cheese Tortellini is 330 calories, but you ate two cups worth, don't write down that you ate 330 calories because that's just not true. You have to be honest with yourself. If you track your calories accurately, this program works amazingly well. When you're at home, you can pull out your measuring cups and scales. When you're out, you pay attention to portion size and make the best educated guess.

Another important thing to consider is that most of us are creatures of habit. We tend to eat the same foods and go to the same restaurants. Once you know how many calories there are in your favorite dishes, you'll always have that stored in your favorites. And when you do go out to a new place, just look up the calories online. Overtime and without even trying, you'll start to develop an encyclopedic knowledge of the calories in different foods.

Tracking your calories is definitely a new habit, but before long you'll be really good at it. One of the most important parts to being successful on this program is to plan out your meals for the next day the night before. I repeat—plan out your meals ahead of time. And if what you eat changes, you just update your calorie tracker accordingly. Always plan ahead, but be flexible. Remember, counting your calories is really a small price to pay for getting to eat whatever you want.

CHAPTER 8

THE ART OF CHOOSING WHAT YOU EAT

Pain is inevitable. Suffering is optional.

—Buddhist Proverb

As an enlightened dieter, the next part to mastering weight loss is the art of choosing what you eat. While it is true that you can lose weight eating whatever you want as long as you stick to your calorie budget, you'll come to find that how you choose to spend those calories will make all the difference. In the last chapter, we discussed how budgeting your calories is similar to budgeting your finances. This same kind of concept also applies when it comes to getting more bang for your buck or for your calorie.

If you are a serious shopper, you probably already know the different strategies for getting the items you want cheaper; such as purchasing during a sale, using coupons, shopping at a discount warehouse, shopping online, or even buying the same items but without the brand name. With a little resourcefulness, there are many smart ways to make your money go further while still getting what you want. This same philosophy works for calories too. While there aren't coupon calories per say, there are ways to get a lot more value for your calories.

In fact, there is an entire art to choosing what you eat that can make weight loss significantly easier. While most dieters are complaining about being hungry, following uninspiring meal plans, or having to rely on willpower—you can have more food than you'll know what to do with. The bottom line is that you do need to consume fewer calories to lose weight, but you don't need to suffer while doing so.

It's important to understand that not all foods are created equal. Certain foods are more filling than others, despite their calorie amounts. Certain foods have more calories than others, despite their portion size. So if you focus on foods that are higher in volume, but lower in calories then you'll get to eat a lot more food for the same amount of calories. If you remember one thing from this chapter, remember that just because you're watching your calories, doesn't mean you need to eat less food.

While the concept of getting more bang for your calorie is the premise of this chapter and will transform the way you diet, it's also important to consider that if you don't like what you eat, you're not going to stick to it long-term. That's why even though you could choose to eat insane amounts of brussels sprouts, egg whites, and tofu all day—for relatively little calories—I wouldn't recommend it unless you truly enjoy those things. In order for this program to work, you must like what you eat.

The trick is to figure out what type of foods you enjoy, and then come up with ways to get more value for your calorie. With a little research, creativity, and planning, there should be no reason why you can't eat a lot of delicious food while still staying within your calorie budget. But before we discuss which foods can help you with this, I want to share with you some examples that might change the way you think about calories.

Example 1:

Let's say in one hand, I have an entire pineapple, and in the other hand, I have one slice of Starbucks's Banana Walnut Bread. The pineapple , which is about as big as my head, has about 450 calories and 12.7 grams of fiber; that's about 50 percent of your daily fiber requirement. The slice of banana bread, which is smaller than a napkin, has about 490 calories and 4 grams of fiber. While both are delicious and healthy, which one do you think will be more filling? Obviously the entire pineapple will be more filling and take much longer to eat. Both have a similar amount of calories, but a very different portion size.

Example 2:

What about this scenario for breakfast? Did you know that for 620 calories you could either eat one Cinnamon Chip Scone from Panera Bread, or for less calories all of the following—two cups of Cheerios with ½ cup 2-Percent Milk (285 calories), one light English muffin with two tablespoons of whipped cream cheese (150 calories), one Nutrigrain Low-Fat

Eggo Waffle (70 calories), and one medium banana (100 calories). See it's not the amount of calories you are given; it's what you choose to do with them.

Example 3:

If you like French toast you might not realize that three slices of your favorite breakfast dish typically has a total of 500 calories. Plus, add ¼ cup of generic brand original syrup and that's another 210 calories. Did you know you could create essentially the same french toast breakfast, but with the following ingredients—three slices of 45-calorie wheat bread (135 calories), plus two eggs (140 calories), and zero calorie coconut oil cooking spray for a total of 275 calories. Plus, use a sugar-free, light calorie version of syrup for only 30 calories per ¼ cup. That's roughly 305 calories versus 710 calories.

Example 4:

On the way to work you could stop by Dunkin Donuts for breakfast and grab a Bacon, Egg & Cheese Bagel (460 calories) or you could order the following— Egg & Cheese Wake-Up Wrap (150 calories) and Hash Browns (200 calories) for only 350 calories. You could even add a glazed Munchkin to your order, and you'd still be consuming fewer calories than the first option.

Example 5:

If you were going to Einstein Bros. Bagels for breakfast, you could order the Spinach & Bacon Egg Panini (770 calories) or the Bagel Thin Egg White Southwest Turkey Sausage Sandwich (350 calories).

Both options are filling and similar in taste, but one is half the amount of calories as the other.

Example 6:

Let's say you were going to stop by Einstein Bros. Bagels and bring something home for an early dinner with 800 calories left. You could order the Turkey Club Panini (800 calories) or all of the following —Bagel Thin Tuscan Chicken Pesto Sandwich (340 calories), Chicken Noodle Soup (120 calories), Potatoe Salad (160 calories), and Fruit and Yogurt Parfait (170 calories). Talk about getting more bang for your calorie!

Example 7:

You could go to Subway and get the 12-inch Chicken Parmesan Sub (1,020 calories), plus a Doritos Package (260 calories), and a 21 oz. Fuze Raspberry Tea (150 calories) for a total for 1,430 calories. Or you could order the following items for only 745 calories— 12-inch Subway Turkey Sandwich (560 calories), Baked Doritos Package (170 calories), and a 21 oz. Minute Maid Light Lemonade (15 calories). Portion wise, you are eating almost identical meals; however, the second option has almost 700 fewer calories.

Example 8:

You could go to McDonald's for lunch and order the Angus Bacon & Cheeseburger (790 calories) and medium fries (380 calories) for a total of 1,170 calories. Or you could get a Grilled Chipotle Barbecue Snack Wrap (250 calories), medium fries (380 calories), side salad (20 calories), and Apple Slices (15 calories) for a total of 665 calories. Interestingly enough, both options would probably put you at the same level of feeling full. The difference is with the second option you're consuming about half the calories; which means that's more calories you're going to get for dinner.

Example 9:

If McDonald's isn't your thing, let's take a trip to Burger King. Did you know that for the same calories in one Texas Double Whopper Sandwich (1,040 calories), you could easily eat five plain hamburgers (220 calories each) or 3 ½ cheeseburgers (270 calories each). Talk about more bang for your beef! Honesty, you'd be much better off ordering a cheeseburger (270 calories), along with 4-piece chicken nuggets (170 calories), value onion rings (150 calories), and fresh apple slices (30 calories) for a total of 620 calories. See, no one said you couldn't eat fast food while on a diet.

Example 10:

Now let's say you really wanted to bring home the Chicken & Shrimp Pesto Cream Penne pasta dish from California Pizza Kitchen (1,370 calories). You could either order takeout from the restaurant or make an identical meal at home for fewer calories. For example you could make the same dish using 1-1/2 cups of penne pasta (528 calories), five medium shrimp (30 calories), three ounces of grilled chicken breast (140 calories), three tablespoons of homemade pesto (240 calories), and two tablespoons of country crock butter (90 calories). This recipe would likely be the same portion size, but it would be around only 1,000 calories instead of 1,370.

Example 11:

Let's say you only have 600 calories left for dinner, but you're really hungry. You could swing by Sbarro and pick up a dish of Chicken Parmigiana with Spaghetti (1,160 calories), and eat half tonight and half tomorrow. Or you could make the following pasta pasta recipe for only 600 calories—2 cups of Farfalle bowtie pasta (400 calories), two sliced All-Natural Chicken Strips (120 calories), ½ cup Organic Garlic Roasted Tomato Sauce (60 calories), ½ cup of chopped red tomatoes (15 calories), 1 tablespoon of minced garlic (5 calories), ½ teaspoon of Kosher salt, and ½ teaspoon of black pepper (0 calories).

Example 12:

Let's say you're having dinner at Pizzaria Uno Chicago Grill. Perhaps, a friend of yours—who isn't an enlightened dieter, but is trying to lose weight—might order the Honey Crisp Chicken Salad without realizing it's 1,320 calories. On the other hand, you might choose to order what you really want for only 810 calories —Uno Breadstick (160 calories), Tomato Soup (180 calories), and the half Mediterranean Traditional Crust Pizza (470 calories). Your meal is likely more filling and delicious than your friend's dinner, and it's 510 calories less!

Example 13:

If you go to your local Mexican restaurant, such as Qdoba, you could easily find a chicken and cheese quesadilla for 1,000 calories. But let's say you only have 650 calories left for dinner that night, you might be better off ordering the three tacos option with grilled chicken, lettuce, and shredded cheese (630 calories). Or you could always go to Chipotle instead and order the Large Chicken and Cheese Quesadilla for 610 calories —remember different ingredients, different calories. Lastly, you could also go home and make your own version of the same beloved dish. For example, take two Mission brand Carb Balance Whole Wheat tortillas (220 calories), three ounces of grilled chicken (192 calories), and ½ cup of shredded Part Skim Mozzarella cheese (160 calories)—all for less than 600 calories.

Example 14:

If you really like pizza like me, you could visit your local pizzeria and order two slices of cheese pizza for roughly 600 calories. You could also order a few slices of pizza marinara for less calories. But another alternative you could do is create your own pizza at home. Take two large FlatOut thin pizza crusts (120 calories each), ½ cup of garlic-roasted tomato sauce (60 calories), 1 cup of shredded lowfat mozzarella cheese (160 calories), and 2 tablespoons of fresh garlic (10 calories). You see, you can create your own delicious and filling pizza flatbreads for a total of only 470 calories. Pizza is a great example of a food that can be made unhealthy or extremely healthy, as well high calorie or low calorie.

Example 15:

Are you in the mood for dessert? Did you know that if you went to the Cheesecake Factory, you could either get one slice of Adam's Peanut Buttercup Fudge Ripple Cheesecake (1,330 calories) or order 12 goblets of fresh strawberries (110 calories each). You could also order the Hot Fudge Sundae (1,530 calories) or more than five dishes of ice cream (280 calories each). Interestingly, I'm sure that one dish of Cheesecake Factory ice cream could more than satisfy your dessert fix.

Example 16:

For all my super healthy eaters, this example is for you. You could order a Starbucks Double Chocolate Chunk Brownie for roughly 500 calories, or instead try making the glutten-free, flourless chocolate zucchini brownie recipe from the skinnytaste.com website. Not only is it way fewer calories, but you would be shocked at how delicious it tastes!

Example 17:

Sticking with the dessert theme, did you know you could either eat one slice of homemade Key Lime Pie (450 calories) or all of the following for only 235 calories —one cup of Honey Dew (60 calories), one sliced up kiwi fruit (45 calories), one Snack Pack Vanilla pudding cup (100 calories), and two Nabisco Graham Crackers (30 calories). With the second option, you're essentially satisfying the same taste buds as the Key Lime Pie. The difference is that it's significantly fewer calories and much healthier.

Example 18:

Here's an example that might make you rethink drinking your calories. For the calories in sixteen ounces of Motts Apple Juice (240 calories), you could eat one medium green apple (95 calories), one Eat Smart Apple Fruit Bar (85 calories), and ½ cup apple sauce (50 calories). Or you could eat an entire Caramel Apple covered with nuts. And if you're both thirsty and hungry, for the same amount of calories as the apple juice, you could eat six Edy's Strawberry Fruit Bars (40 calories each).

Example 19:

If you're going to the movies and want to have a snack you might want to rethink visiting the concession stand. Forget the prices! Did you know that one large size popcorn at AMC Movie Theaters is over 1,000 calories? Instead, you could order a small popcorn (630 calories) or large soft pretzel (480 calories). Or you could bring your own snacks and have Trader Joe's Kettle Popcorn package (110 calories) and a Snack Well's Pretzels Pack (110 calories) for a total of 220 calories.

Example 20:

If you're used to eating a lot of sweets, you might be surprised to find that eating fruit can satisfy many of the same cravings. For example, you could have one package of Peanut M&Ms (250 calories) or the following snack—prepare one cup of apple slices (95 calories) with one tbsp of peanut butter (95 calories). For 190 calories, you can satisfy your sweet tooth and eat alot more food in the process. Similarly, swap a Strawberry Flavored Twizzlers package (250 calories) for 1½ cups of strawberries (75 calories) with ½ cup of Cool Whip (100 calories). For only 175 calories you'll have a delicious and filling snack. It's not just about making healthier choices; it's about getting creative and getting more for your calories.

Hopefully these examples help illustrate the point that I'm trying to make—which is that it's not the calories that limit you, but your food choices. The bottom line is that if you find yourself still feeling hungry throughout the day, then you're not getting enough value for your calories. This diet isn't about swapping junk food for salad, or carbs for protein; rather it's about determining what you like to eat and then figuring out how to make those calories go further. Plus, you might discover some new and delicious foods along the way that can deliver a lot of bang for their calorie.

While I encourage you to eat the types of things you like, you may also want to consider not wasting your calories on things you're not that into. Meaning, if it's the weekend and you love dessert then you may want to have a lower calorie entree, and spend those calories on an awesome dessert. If you're like me and don't care about dessert, you may want to spend your calories on your entrée, but skip dessert. Personally, I like to think of using calories like spending money. Don't just spend money for the sake of spending money. Be smart and spend your calories wisely.

I'm not trying to say that you shouldn't order your favorite high-calorie dishes. If you really want to eat something then consciously make the choice to fit it into your calorie budget. After all, nothing is off limits and it's your choice. However, if most of the time you strive to eat foods that can give you a lot more bang for your calorie, you'll find you're able to eat so much more food. Plus, knowing how to get more for less calories helps accommodate those times when you do want to have your favorite high-calorie dish.

As an enlightened dieter, you don't need to change what you like, instead just get creative. Choose something similar for fewer calories, or swap the ingredients for lower calorie alternatives. You don't have to sacrifice taste or portion size just because you're following a calorie budget. At this point in your life, you like what you like. While you may be open to making healthier choices and trying new food, you're taste and preferences are already set. That being said, if you want weight loss and maintenance to be easy, then eat the sorts of foods you like and will go back to eating once you reach your dream weight.

Now let's get something straight—I'm not in any way encouraging you to eat fast-food every day if you like Burger King a lot. While you can still visit the king from time to time, what I want you to do is think about what types of foods you like because you can make these same types of foods at home. You can pretty much take any menu item, find out the ingredients, and create your own recipe that's healthier and for fewer calories.

For example, if you like chicken strips and French fries take a trip to the frozen food section at WholeFoods. Here you'll find organic, non-gmo chicken strips that are low in calories and taste great.

You might also find crinkle cut French fries or Sweet Potato French fries that are healthy, taste amazing, and won't blow your calorie budget. Now I'm not trying to push these healthier alternatives , but some of them taste so good that if you dressed them up in fast-food packaging, you wouldn 't even be able to tell the difference.

Here's a great example. In 2010, Taco Bell came out with the Beefy Crunch Burrito (510 calories) for a limited-time. While I don't often eat at fast-food restaurants, I definitely made an exception for this particular burrito—a flour tortilla with ground beef, rice, nacho cheese sauce, reduced-fat sour cream, and Flamin' Hot Fritos. However, shortly after my discovery of this item, they stopped serving it.

Instead of starting a letter-writing campaign to petition for it back or driving to other states to find it, I decided to try and create my own version of it at home. Well I'm kidding about the driving to other states.

In all seriousness, I took an eight-inch low-calorie flour tortilla (80 calories), ⅓ cup of extra lean ground beef (100 calories), ⅓ cup of brown rice (60 calories), ¼ cup Nacho Cheese Dip (40 calories), two tablespoons of light sour cream (40 calories), and eight Fritos Original Corn Chips (40). Since I couldn't find the Flamin' Hot Fritos version, I just dipped the chips in hot sauce for no additional calories. Not only was I able to make almost an identical dish, but also I was able to do so for 150 calories less. In addition, I even came up with a delicious grilled chicken version for even fewer calories.

Funny enough, Taco Bell has since brought back the infamous Beefy Crunch Burrito, but under the moniker "Beefy Nacho Loaded Griller"—same burrito, but a smaller size and for only 420 calories. A small victory for burrito lovers everywhere! While I'll still venture to Taco Bell now and then for my favorite item, it's nice to know that I can always make a healthier version at home and for fewer calories. Remember, with a little ingenuity and resourcefulness, you can find almost any recipe online and customize it to meet your needs.

Today, there are so many low-calorie alternatives available. Like in the Subway example above, you can choose the Regular Doritos Individual package (260 calories) or the Baked Doritos Individual package (170 calories). Both taste great, but one is approximately 100 calories less. Another great example can be found when you're shopping for bread. For instance, if you're looking for bread, you might find one brand that has forty calories per slice and another brand that has a hundred calories per slice; both with the same amount of fiber. It's kind of like buying a Marc Jacobs bag at T.J. Max; you're getting the same thing, but for a fraction of the cost.

Now you don't always need to choose the lower-calorie alternative to have success. Sometimes you just might want to swap one of the ingredients. For example, you don't have to substitute scrambled eggs for egg whites and bacon for turkey bacon. But you might compromise and make a breakfast sandwich with one bagel thin (110 calories), one scrambled egg (70 calories), and one slice of turkey bacon (30 calories).

Or, you may choose to substitute egg whites for whole eggs that day so you don't use your additional "mad money" calories. It's all about spending your calories on the items that are important to you.

While the art of choosing what you eat is definitely about finding lower calorie alternatives for your favorite foods, it's also about discovering new foods that can help make your calories go further. In my experience there are certain foods you can incorporate—such as fruit, vegetables, whole grains, and protein-rich foods — that will give you a lot of bang for your calorie and help keep you full. You don't need to eat these foods to lose weight, but you'll find that many of these items will make your calories go further.

Personally, I'm constantly eating fruits such as strawberries, raspberries, blackberries, blueberries, apples, melons, and mangos. In my opinion, fruits are some of nature's most delicious foods. I eat lots of fruit because I think they taste great and I can eat a lot of them for relatively little calories. Fruits are packed with fiber and are high in water content so they're quite filling for their calorie content. So if you want to add food that delivers a lot of value, try incorporating a few servings of fruit per day.

If for some reason the thought of fruit doesn't get you excited, there are a few tricks you can do to make it more enticing. For example, add a packet of Truvia sugar to a bowl of blackberries and it'll taste like candy. Add cool whip to a bowl of strawberries and it'll taste like heaven. Add a bit of peanut butter or honey to your apple slices and it'll serve as a tasty and filling dessert.

Add banana slices to your bowl of cereal, raspberries to your oatmeal, or blueberries to your pancakes and make your meal more delicious and filling.

Now when it comes to vegetables, I have to admit that I'm really not a fan. However, since many vegetables have so little calories for their mass, I've learned a few tricks over the years to make them more enjoyable. Dip raw broccoli, baby carrots, or celery into ranch dressing. Take baby spinach and sauté it in garlic and olive oil. Stir-fry baby corn, broccoli, and noodles in soy sauce. Add lettuce and cucumbers to a sandwich to give it more mass. While I'm not a fan of beans, add them to a plate of rice and you'll have a perfectly nutritious and filling meal.

When it comes to fruits and vegetables, you can add them to your meals or eat them in-between meals as a filling snack. If you don't already eat them, you might be surprised how good they can taste. Remember, just like any other food, you still need to check the calories. If you focus on the items that are low in calories and high in volume, you'll get to eat a lot more for the same calories. So try different fruits and vegetables, and incorporate the ones you like.

Now there is absolutely nothing wrong with eating white bread, pasta, or rice. While there isn't as much nutritional value, it won't make you gain weight and typically has the same amount of calories as the multigrain, wheat, or brown alternatives. However, one thing to consider is that because the latter usually has more fiber and is slower to digest, you might need to eat less of it to make you feel full. So experiment and try multigrain bread instead of white bread, wheat pasta instead of white pasta, and brown rice instead of white rice. If you don't like it then go back to the original. On the other hand, it might become an acquired taste and once you get used to it, you might actually prefer it.

Remember, it's not all or nothing. For example, when it comes to sushi I always get white rice instead of brown rice. When it comes to pasta dishes, I typically make the wheat version instead of the white. When it comes to cereals, I prefer the whole grain cereals to the overly processed and refined ones. When it comes to bread, it depends on what I'm eating. I usually like my bagels with white bread, my sandwiches with wheat bread, and my tortillas made from corn. Be open to trying whole-grain alternatives, but also eat what you like and what keeps you feeling good.

Another great food to add to your meals is protein. When it comes to protein, it doesn't take that much of it to make you feel full. For example, you'd get full way faster eating a petite 6 oz. filet mignon than eating a bowl of chips. That's why I often add eggs to my breakfast or add chicken to my homemade personal pizza or pasta dishes. Whether its meat, poultry, seafood, eggs, beans, tofu, or other protein-rich foods, add it to your meals to fill you up and make your calories go further. Protein is important for your body, but it's also great for your diet.

Some research suggests that foods high in protein can help control hunger and foods high in fat aren't as filling. While there may be some truth to this, I also think it depends on the particular food and the person.

If you find that certain dishes aren't as satisfying then you may want to not eat them as much. On the other hand, if you find something extremely filling and delicious then you may want to incorporate it more often. Overall, I wouldn't make anything entirely off limits, but make wise choices and focus on the foods that will keep you satisfied.

Again, when it comes to fruit, vegetables, whole-grains, and protein-rich foods, these are just recommendations. In my experience, these are the foods that will help make weight loss easier because they taste good and are filling. However, just like people have different taste, different foods can affect people differently. That's why it's important to try new foods and experiment, and don't forget to check the calories.

Just like there are certain foods that will give you more bang for your calorie, there are other items that are empty calories and may not be worth it. For example, drinking a 12 fl. oz. can of regular Coca Cola will not make you feel full, but it will cost you 140 calories. Instead, you could drink water, sparkling water, or unsweetened iced tea for zero calories. If you want to spend your calories on soda drinks and juices that's totally fine, but just remember you could be eating those calories.

If you're making smart choices and focusing on getting more value for your calorie, there is no reason you should feel hungry while sticking to your calorie budget. If you're not feeling good and satisfied throughout the day then you 're not doing this program right!

Mastering the art of choosing what you eat doesn't happen overnight. It's a learning process, so be patient with yourself as you learn, discover and get more creative. You might eat something that left you feeling hungry and unsatisfied, and decide not to order that again. Or you might cook something that was super filling and delicious, and start making that a regular part of your meal plan. Remember, just because you have to eat fewer calories, doesn't mean you need to eat less food. Focus on the foods that you love, the ones that fill you up and that pack a lot of bang for their calorie, and it won't even feel like you're on a diet.

CHAPTER 9
HOW TO LISTEN TO YOUR BODY

> We have two ears and one mouth, so that we
> can listen twice as much as we speak.
>
> —Epictetus

It can also be said that we have two ears and one mouth, so that we can listen twice as much as we eat. Part of the secret to weight control is learning how to listen to your body when it comes to eating. Unfortunately, many of us have tuned out these natural cues over the years. But, if you pay close attention, your body will tell you exactly when to eat and when to stop. Learning how to get in touch with these signals can be one of your greatest tools for mastering weight loss and maintenance.

If you think about it, hunger and perfect weight control are intrinsic parts of nature. I mean how many overweight animals do you see in the wild? Not many. I read this great article titled "Why Don't Animals Get Fat?" It made me laugh as the author asked, "When was the last time you saw an obese orangutan. Or a llama with love handles?"[21] But it's true.

As the author points out, "Wild animals are experts at keeping in damned good shape without ever forcing themselves to eat less and exercise more." In fact, the only time you ever see animals become obese are when they are domesticated.[22] So what is it about wild animals that make them maintain this balance naturally?

The standard explanation is that animals have to work hard to get their food, so they stay thin. But as the author points out, many times this just isn't the case. For example, male lions typically lounge around for twenty hours a day while the female lions do most of the hunting. They sit back, relax, and chow down on high-calorie zebra meat.[23] Yet despite this posh lifestyle, male lions still remain lean and slim. While they might not do all the hunting, they still have to defend the pride.

What about other wild animals such as herbivores that don't have to work that hard for their food? Have you ever seen a mountain goat stalk and then hunt grass? My point exactly! It's typically a twenty-four-hour grass buffet, yet mountain goats don't eat themselves into a food coma. Wild animals instinctively know how much to eat in order to stay strong and trim, so they can outrun their predators. In their native environments, animals just don't get overweight. They eat what they need and they don't overindulge.

This article explains it well, "In animals, increases or decreases in the availability of food don't lead to weight gain or loss, they lead to more offspring. In other words, when animals have easy access to food, they don't get fat, they get freaky!" Additionally, "the lack of observed fluctuation in body composition of animals throughout periods of fast and famine suggest that, instead of trying to acquire as big of a caloric surplus as possible, they live in equilibrium with their environment, weathering times of both feast and famine with their health and fitness intact."[24]

So are humans the exception to the animal kingdom? I don't think so, at least not naturally. While there are many differences that separate us from animals, knowing when to eat and when to stop shouldn't be one of them. If you think about it, many of us aren't that different from male lions. So we're not nocturnal, but we typically sit at a desk all day, at home we lounge around, and we often have access to high-calorie meals. The difference is an obese lion wouldn't last long in the wild.

For humans, it's much easier and socially acceptable to become overweight. We don't have to worry about hunting our meals or defending our pride. We also have access to a larger variety of food and live in an age where dining is entertainment. However, that doesn't mean overeating and becoming overweight is natural for humans. Overindulging and binge-eating are learned and adopted behaviors. Plus, obesity is an unnatural state for the human body. It's ironic; the point of eating is to stay alive, yet if you abuse it, obesity can kill you.

It doesn't matter if you are as active as a cheetah or inactive as a sleuth. I know very active individuals who are on the chubby side and very inactive individuals who are thin. The more active we are the more energy we use, but even if we aren't very active it doesn't mean we need to be overweight. Wherever you fall on the spectrum, you can still be thin through consuming the right amount of calories and listening to your body.

Throughout the world, there are plenty of countries that celebrate food and are exposed to high-calorie meals; nevertheless, they remain naturally slim. But when it comes to the United States the difference seems to be the mindset and behavior surrounding food. There is nothing wrong with enjoying food and choosing delicious meals. However, the difference is that most of the world eats to live and not lives to eat.

One of the reasons why so many Americans struggle with weight control is that somewhere along the line they stopped paying attention to their bodies' natural signals. While most of us don't live in the wild, these natural cues are still there; we just need to learn how to pay attention.

It's important to understand that humans eat for one of two reasons: hunger and appetite. While these two may seem synonymous and can overlap in terms of weight control, they actually mean very different things. Hunger is the physiological need for food. Appetite, on the other hand, is the desire for, or interest in food without a physiological need; it's a psychological response.[25]

Keep in mind, the difference between hunger and appetite doesn't necessarily affect what you eat, rather it affects when you eat and how much you eat of it. That's why learning to distinguish between the two can help you learn to eat the way nature intended. Imagine eating what you want, whenever you're hungry, but never binge-eating or overindulging. Learning to listen to your body can help make weight loss easier and maintenance easy.

Hunger is an instinctive, protective mechanism that helps your body function and keep you alive. So when you start to feel hungry, it's actually a good thing; it means it's time to eat and you should listen. If you pay close attention to hunger and eat accordingly, your body will reward you with high-energy, increased focus, and an overall good feeling. If you choose to ignore hunger you'll feel weak, famished, and ultimately it will control you.

Think of your body like your car's gas tank and hunger like the gauge. The gas light just doesn't turn on out of nowhere. There is a spectrum you can see as you start to run low on fuel. It's the same thing with your body. There is a spectrum of symptoms you will experience as you start to run low on energy—all the way from starving to hungry to satisfied to stuffed. And just like you wouldn't tell your car to suck it up if you were running out of gas, you shouldn't do the same with your body.

Your body will let you know it's time to eat with subtle signals and cues. At first, you'll notice a slight physiological urge to eat. This is a good time to get ready to eat soon or to have a light snack. If you don't do anything, then your body will kick it up a notch with hunger pangs and an overall empty feeling. When you experience this, your body is letting you know it needs food.

If still you don't eat anything, eventually you'll end up feeling ravenously hungry, extremely weak, headachy, light-headed, and possibly irritable. It's where the saying "I'm so hungry, I could eat a horse" comes from. If you can, you never want to let yourself get to this extreme stage of hunger. While the symptoms can vary from person to person, what you will notice is that when it comes to hunger, it's physical, and it won't be a question because you'll know you're hungry.

Not listening to your body and letting yourself get to the point of starving can be dangerous for dieters. The hungrier you let yourself become, the more willpower you will need to make smart choices. Interestingly enough, when it comes to intense hunger pangs it doesn't take much food to make the pain go away. Believe it or not, a few crackers or a small fruit can usually do the trick. The problem is when most people get ravenously hungry they make poor choices and don't know when to stop; these are the times when people often overindulge.

While it may seem like common sense to ignore or try and control hunger while trying to lose weight, in reality the opposite is true. A constantly satisfied belly will keep you thin. Whereas an empty stomach will make you feel physically and mentally weak. Remember, the better you feel, the easier weight loss becomes.

Your body is naturally efficient at letting you know when it's time to eat. While most people rely on a clock to tell them when to eat, you don't always have to. For example, if you are having lunch at 12:30 p.m., but you find yourself getting really hungry by noon then listen to your body and eat earlier. If for some reason you can't change your mealtime, then have a low-calorie snack to hold you over until your next meal.

My rule is that whenever you are legitimately hungry, you should always eat. That doesn't mean you need to eat something high in calories. Even when you are sticking to a calorie budget, it's easy to choose low-calorie options that won't interfere with your calories. If you ever find yourself in a situation where you don't have any calories left for the day, but you are really hungry, you can always go the vegetable route. Cucumbers and celery are examples of vegetables that have almost no calories, but will fill you up.

Trust me, when you're that hungry, it doesn't matter what you eat; you just need food to give you energy and make the hunger pangs go away. Make your best effort to keep yourself satisfied throughout the day, but if you notice yourself feeling extremely hungry, make sure you listen and eat. It's a mistake to not listen to your body when it's trying to tell you that you need food. So when hunger calls, pick up!

Unlike hunger, appetite is the psychological desire for or interest in food. It can be triggered by seeing or smelling something that looks delicious. Even if you are not hungry, you can still have an appetite. For example, let's say you already ate a filling lunch, but then you smell Chinese food in the next cubicle, and all of a sudden you want some. Or let's say you wake up hungry in the middle of the night, and you know that one cookie could satisfy you, but instead you finish off the entire tub of ice cream.

Another good way to explain the difference between appetite and hunger is if you're hungry, a few slices of pizza will probably be enough to satisfy you. However, it's your appetite that will make you go for seconds and perhaps finish the entire pie even though you're already full. You know that popular saying that your eyes are bigger than your stomach—well that's where appetite comes in.

When you feel the urge to eat something because it looks or smells good, but you recognize you are not actually hungry, you'll find yourself at an important crossroad. First, acknowledge that you aren't physiologically hungry, so you don't need to eat. Second, realize that you can always eat that item tomorrow.

If you really want something, but don't have room in your calorie budget, a little technique that I do is this— don't eat it now, but make sure you eat it tomorrow, and fit it into your calories. This way you're not saying no, you're just delaying when you are going to eat it. You might wakeup the next morning, and not even want it anymore. But if you do, definitely make you sure you incorporate it into your daily plan.

The problem with focusing on appetite instead of listening to hunger is that it can lead to overeating and emotional eating. Since food can provide pleasure, many people have learned to satisfy psychological cravings with food. Think about times when you've indulged for whatever reason and it had nothing to do with actual hunger. Treating emotional or psychological issues with food can lead to eating disorders.

Some people eat for entertainment, for pleasure, or out of boredom. Others eat when they are sad or depressed, to try and make themselves feel better. Some people overeat when they are stressed, and others when they are happy. In fact, some dieters overeat as punishment when they believe they messed up on their diet. Then their subsequent behavior becomes a self-fulfilling prophecy. Whatever the reason is, when food is used as a crutch or a coping mechanism, it creates an unhealthy relationship.

Think about this, when you rely on hunger and then you eat, the hunger goes away and you know when to stop. But, if you eat for emotional reasons, such as feeling sad, eating doesn't take sadness away, so then, how do you know when to stop? You don't and you keep eating. While emotional eating may provide a fleeting gratification, after you're finished eating, the emotional emptiness still remains.

There is a line from the movie *The Fat Boy Chronicles* that always stuck with me. It says "I didn't know how to deal with the pain, so I would eat. I would eat when I was happy, and I would eat when I was sad. I would eat when I was bored. But no matter what, I was always left feeling empty."

I'm also reminded of the character Fat Bastard from the Austin Powers movie who said, "I eat because I'm unhappy, and I'm unhappy because I eat. It's a vicious cycle." Unfortunately, this is a reality for many people who struggle with their weight and deal with their problems by eating.

So how do you free yourself from the bondage of emotional eating? You learn to listen to your body and eat the way nature intended. That means you always eat when you are hungry and never eat when you are not hungry. You learn to distinguish between hunger and appetite or between physiological hunger and psychological hunger. Again, this doesn't really affect what you eat; it more affects when you eat and how much you eat. If you learn how to listen to your body and eat accordingly, you'll develop a natural and healthy relationship with food.

If you ever feel the emotional urge to eat, but recognize you are not actually hungry, it's important to identify what is the cause for that feeling. Are you bored, tired, sad, stressed, or disappointed? By doing this you can identify the issue, recognize you don't need to eat, and think of how you want to replace this urge with another activity or solution.

For example, if you're feeling bored or need entertainment, you can watch a movie, read a book, play a video game, or watch a YouTube video. If you're looking for pleasure, you can go get a massage, get a manicure, or do some online shopping! If you are sad or had a bad day, you can listen to uplifting music, exercise or treat yourself to something special and rewarding that doesn't involve food. Especially when you are feeling stressed, exercise is a great way to deal with all that energy. Whatever the reason is, there is always an alternative activity you can do that would be just as satisfying without the calories.

Overeating and overindulging have practically become the norm in the United States. In fact, the way we think about being full is very different from many countries. My husband is Brazilian and always corrects me to say that I'm satisfied, instead of full. In Brazil, it's not polite to say you are full; you're supposed to say you're satisfied. Using the world "full" is just a choice of vocabulary, but he's completely right when it comes to this attitude. There is a big difference between being full/satisfied and full/stuffed.

In the United States, most people eat until they are full or stuffed. But when I talk about being full in this book, I'm talking about full or satisfied. When you eat until you are satisfied, at the end of a meal you feel great. You are no longer hungry, your stomach feels better, and you have increased energy. On the other hand, when you overeat, at the end of the meal you actually feel bad. You'll likely feel tired, lethargic, and even discomfort.

If you think about it, eating too much is actually a very uncomfortable feeling. We've all been there. If you've had to undo your pants at a restaurant or let out a belch to not be in pain, you've eaten way too much food. Not only is eating like this uncomfortable, but if you continuously do this, it will stretch out your stomach over time. That means, that it will take more and more food to make you feel that level of stuffed. If you continue to overeat and stretch out your stomach, you will continue to gain weight.

I think that's why a lot of diets suggest eating smaller meals and more frequently throughout the day to retrain your body to stop overeating. However, how often you want to eat is really up to you as long as you listen to your body. My suggestion is to have three meals throughout the day, and fill in the gaps with snacks if you're feeling hungry.

Just like your body subtly lets you know when it's time to eat, if you listen to your body, it will also tell you when you should stop. While you're eating you might notice yourself starting to get a little full. This is a good time to take a rest and reevaluate in a few minutes. If you're still hungry, eat more; but if you feel good and satisfied, then you should stop.

You must learn to retrain yourself that full means satisfied and not stuffed. For many people, this is one of the biggest adjustments. And since you're allowed to eat whenever you are actually hungry, you can stop when you're full without any concern.

They key to paying attention to your body and not overeating comes down to one thing—eating slowly. I can't emphasize enough how important it is to take your time and eat slow. Typically, you probably scarf down your food, and don't allow your brain to catch up to your stomach. When you do this, you'll likely eat until your plate is empty or until you're in physical discomfort. Eating shouldn't be a race to the finish line. Instead, take your time, eat slowly, and savor the taste. Not only will you enjoy your meal more, but also, you'll allow your body to naturally let you know you when you're satisfied.

Unfortunately, you can't trust plate and portion size in this day and age. But just because portions everywhere are getting larger, doesn't mean that you need to. When I go out to restaurants, I often find myself not being able to finish the plate. Depending on the restaurant, sometimes I can barely eat half of it. Instead of pushing myself to eat everything, I stop when I'm full and satisfied. In fact, I've even stopped with just a few bites away from finishing my plate because I didn't want to overextend my stomach.

Now some of us were raised with the notion that you should always finish your plate because kids in other countries are starving. It's a nice concept, but I'm sure you've realized by now that whether you finish your plate or not, it isn't going to affect world hunger. I would never encourage anyone to waste food, but you also shouldn't keep eating when you're not hungry. If you can't finish your plate, let someone else finish it or take it home.

Naturally thin people know how to do this really well. Because they can eat whatever they want and whenever they are hungry, they don't feel the need to overeat. Next time you are out at a restaurant, eat slowly, eat what you need to be satisfied, and don't overindulge. You'll feel much better at the end of the meal. Remember, it's not the last supper! You can always eat again in a few hours, if you're legitimately hungry. When you listen to your body, it will reward you—you'll look great, feel great, and start to develop a healthier relationship with food.

If you can master this concept, you'll learn how to eat like a naturally thin person. The key is to listen to your body. It must become second nature—eat whenever you're hungry and don't eat when you're full.

By combining calorie counting with listening to your body, you'll lose weight naturally, develop a healthy relationship with food, and set yourself up to keep the weight off for good.

CHAPTER 10

HOW TO EAT OUT AND STILL LOSE WEIGHT

A firm free does not fear the storm.

—Indonesian Proverb

Eating out can be one of the most challenging issues for dieters, when it comes to sticking to their calorie goals. Whether you're out at a restaurant, away on vacation or simply eating at someone else's house, there are often more temptations for high-calorie dishes, unknown calorie amounts, and social pressures that can make it more difficult. However, as an enlightened dieter there is no reason to worry. There are a few different strategies you can use to help you eat out and still stick to your plan.

The easiest scenario when it comes to dining out is when you're going to a restaurant that lists its nutritional information online. For example, if you know you're going to Chicago Pizzeria Uno for dinner, you can look up the calorie information on the restaurant's website, pick out what you want to eat ahead of time, and budget your calories for the day accordingly. With a little planning, you can go to your favorite restaurants, while staying perfectly on track with your goals.

Looking up the calories ahead of time is easy to do and can actually be fun. Before you go to a restaurant, spend some time looking at all of your different menu options. For example, you might want to go for the 600 calorie pasta dish, or split up your 600 calories with a soup, appetizer, and lower-calorie entree. You could also choose a higher-calorie meal, but split it with someone along with an appetizer. There are a lot of creative ways to spend your calories.

Plus, if you really want a certain dish that is higher in calories, you could always make sure to eat high-bulk, low-calorie foods for breakfast and lunch to guarantee you'll have enough calories for dinner. With a little planning and creativity, there shouldn't be anything that you can't accommodate.

These days you can find nutritional facts online for almost any restaurant chain. From Burger King to Bertuccis, McDonald's to Maggiano's, and Panda Express to P.F. Chang's, you can look up the calories online ahead of time. Some restaurant websites, such as Qdoba and Chipotle, even have customized nutritional calculators, so that you can personalize your order and know exactly how many calories you'll consume. Even if the restaurant doesn't post the information on its website, with a little research you can usually find it elsewhere online.

Recently, the U.S. Food and Drug Administration (FDA) has issued two proposed regulations that would ensure calorie labeling on menus and menu boards in chain restaurants, retail food establishments, and vending machines with twenty or more locations.[26] This is great news for calorie counters. As time goes on, more and more restaurants will jump on the bandwagon and make their nutrition information available, as well as provide lower-calorie menu alternatives.

The Cheesecake Factory is a prime example of a restaurant with typically high-calorie dishes that came out with an alternative low-calorie menu. We're not talking about sauceless dishes and bunless burgers here. The Cheesecake Factory's Skinnylicious menu has delicious items that are decent in size and stay under 600 calories per plate. From pasta to burgers to tacos and more—they have it all!

Many chain restaurants are starting to offer additional low-calorie menus, or sections of the menu dedicated to low calorie dishes. The clever restaurants, such as The Cheesecake Factory, are realizing that fewer calories don't have to mean smaller portions or boring foods. Whether the calories are listed on the menu itself, or you have to look it up online ahead of time, restaurants that provide this nutritional information are the way to go when you want to eat out and still stick to your calorie budget.

Restaurants are also starting to understand that listing the calories doesn't necessarily deter people from eating there. This is true even at restaurants with notoriously high-calorie dishes. Those that don't care about calories will keep coming anyway. Those that do care about calories can now incorporate their favorite restaurants and dishes into their calorie budget, and still eat out while trying to lose weight.

Another neat thing about eating out at restaurant chains is that the calories listed are usually for the entire plate. That means you can order your meal and enjoy it without measuring or checking portions. However, when checking the nutritional facts, make sure it's for the entire dish. Some restaurants have very high-calorie dishes, and choose to list the calories per serving instead of for the entire plate.

A good rule of thumb is to always check the serving size whether it's on a restaurant's nutritional factsheet, or even on the back of a packaged snack. These days almost all restaurants put the calories for the entire dish, but it's important to keep an eye out for those that don't.

Whether you're going out for breakfast, lunch, or dinner, going to a restaurant that provides its nutritional information makes things easy. But what do you do when you go to a non-chain restaurant that doesn't provide this information? Or perhaps you're not a fan of big chains, and prefer mom-and-pop restaurants.

The good news is that most restaurants, even smaller ones, do put their menus online so you can view them ahead of time. In fact, in this Web 2.0 world, it's hard to find a restaurant that desn't have a website and list its menu online. In these cases, all you need to do is do a little research to look up the general calories for the items you are interested in on the menu. With a little investigating, you can still figure out the approximate calorie amounts. In fact, you can even do all the research you need right from your smartphone without anyone even knowing.

For example, if you're going to a local steakhouse, a six ounce filet mignon will pretty much have the same calories wherever you go. If you're going out for sushi, you can find the general calorie amounts for different rolls online. If you go out for burgers or pizza the same applies. Whether it's a soup, salad, appetizer, entrée, or dessert, if you do your research, you'll have educated information as to what the calories likely are. I've been doing this particular strategy for years with a lot of success.

When doing this type of research there are different online sources you can use to help you. You can use your calorie tracker food database, go to a website like Nutritionix.com, or do a general Google search for calories. Also, something that I like to do is look up a similar meal at a chain restaurant that provides its nutritional information.

For example, if I'm planning on getting a large or dinner size Grilled Chicken Caesar salad at a random restaurant, I can look up that item at Applebee's and see that it's 820 calories there. At Chili's, the same salad is 1,000 calories. Whatever restaurant you go to, a full size Grilled Chicken Caesar Salad will likely be around 900 calories or a little less. You can do this with just about anything. This approach isn't an exact science, but you would be surprised how well it actually works.

Even if you don't have an opportunity to check the calories ahead of time, with smart phones, you can go online and look up the calories. I recall one particular dinner in which I decided to change my meal and was able to check the calories for a different dish before the waitress even came back to take our order. Having the Internet at our fingertips is like having a food oracle at your beck and call.

When dining out, you should always try and stick to your weight loss calorie goal. However, if you really want the extra few hundred calories, you can always dip into your "mad money" or additional calories. Also, remember to spend your calories on foods you really enjoy; don't waste them.

What I'm trying to say here is use your calories wisely. Personally, I'm a French fries snob. I don't eat them that often, so when I do, I'm not going to waste my calories on cold French fries, or on average tasting ones. I'm only going to eat them, if they are really good. How you want to use your calories is completely up to you. My suggestion is that if you are going to go for the high-calorie items, make sure it's on the good stuff.

One issue that seems to resonate with most dieters is whether or not to eat the bread while waiting for their meal. If you want to have a dinner roll then have one, and work it into your calorie budget. There are typically between 150–170 calories per roll. Or you might not be that into bread, and rather use those calories for something else. dy advice is that if you are going to eat the bread, only have on epiece becuase you are going to want to save room for your entrée.

Since you are listening to your body and not overeating, what's the point of filling up on bread when you have a delicious meal coming? Personally, I eat a lot of bread at home, but when it comes to eating out, I usually skip it, or only have one piece. Remember, during the time between placing your order and when your food arrives you are not going to die of starvation. Have patience, and save the room and your calories for the main course!

Another good tip is that when you're going out to eat, don't go starving. For example, if you know you're going out for a late dinner, have a low-caloric but filling snack before you leave. This way, you're not ravenously hungry by the time you get to the restaurant and the food arrives. When your body feels good, you don't need that much willpower; but when you're ravenously hungry, it can be difficult to make good choices. It's like they say—you shouldn't go to grocery store when you're starving. You'll get home and wonder who bought those Twinkies.

While eating out, consider not wasting your calories on regular soda, juice, or alcohol. You'd be surprised to discover how high in calories many of these items actually are. One drink can easily turn into three or four, and that's an extra 200-1,000 calories. If you are determined to incorporate alcohol into your calorie budget, then just make sure you do your research and select the lowest calorie drinks available, and add them to your calorie tracker

According to WebMD, whether you're drinking beer or a cosmo, the higher the alcohol content, the higher the calories. And when it comes to portion size, the average serving size of wine and alcoholic beverages is probably smaller than you think.[27] Also, beware of the dessert drinks such as the Chocolate Martini, or the Strawberry Shortcake Cocktail. You'd faint if you saw how many calories are packed in these drinks. I don't know about you, but I'd rather eat a cheesecake than drink one any day.

While you might find eating out a little more challenging and inflexible than eating at home, you can still be creative with your meals. For example, if you have enough calories for a hamburger, but not for French fries, then order the hamburger, but ask for a side of vegetables or fruit instead. If you need to shave off some calories from an entrée, you can ask for a lighter sauce, or sauce on the side. Keep in mind; you don't need to finish your entire plate. You can always eat half of your meal and pack the other half up to go.

Most of the time while eating out, you should be able to figure out the calories ahead of time; however, there will still be times when you are unable to do so. You might be away on vacation, at an event, or perhaps going to someone's house where you just don't know the calories. There is a different strategy you can use when faced with this type of situation. After all, you don't want counting calories to interfere with your life.

As you start looking up calories and getting familiar with different types of food, you'll inevitably learn which items are low in calories, and which items are not. For example, Caesar salad, while delicious, is typically high in calories. A house salad with balsamic vinaigrette is typically low in calories. Also fish and chicken, when not fried, breaded, or covered with sauce is typically low in calories. Add a white cream sauce to the same dish and the calories will soar.

As part of the researching and calorie counting process, you will start to become good at knowing which foods are lower in calories. You can use this knowledge to consciously make low-calorie choices in situations when you are not able to count your calories. Plus, you can always use your smartphone to look up the general calories in a dish if you aren't sure, and then make the lowest calorie choice.

For those of you who are rolling your eyes, remember that 95 percent of the time you are going to be counting your calories and eating whatever you want. But, the few instances when you are unable to do so, you don't want it to interfere with your weight loss. These are the times when you will focus on choosing low-calorie, but filling foods.

If you are facing a buffet and are unable to count your calories, then you'll want to select the known lower-calorie items. For example, forgo the Rigatoni Vodka pasta that night, and stick with a plain salad with low calorie dressing and grilled chicken. And if you can't stop thinking about Rigatoni Vodka then this is what you do—skip it that night, but make sure the next day you go to your favorite Italian restaurant and fit it into your calories.

If you're going to a wedding or similar event, and they offer you the dinner choices ahead of time, then you may be able to count your calories. But, if you don't know what the options are, then you'll have to make the lowest calorie choice. You can choose the beef, chicken, or fish with a salad, and ask for the sauce on the side. You can also skip dessert at the affair, and instead have a low-calorie dessert when you get home.

Most importantly don't go to the wedding or event hungry. When you feel satisfied, you'll surprise yourself at how easy it is to turn down those pigs in a blanket. When it comes to the cocktail hour, stay away from the fried foods and other high-calorie hors d'oeuvres. You can never go wrong with vegetables and fruit, as they are low in calories and a great way to fill up. If you really want to have a high-calorie item, then allow yourself to have one or two, and then fill the rest of your plate with vegetables.

Now you may run into a situation in which you can't count your calories and a high-calorie option is unavoidable. Let's say you're having dinner at your fiancé's parents' house for the first time, and you don't want to offend them. There will be times, albeit infrequently, when you will just have to eat what you you are served. Don't let the situation be an excuse to indulge or overeat. A really good rule of thumb that I like to use in these types of situations is to use your hand size to measure your portion. It means whatever you eat at one sitting should be no larger than your fist. Also be sure to eat slowly, chew your food thoroughly before swallowing, and take your time and enjoy eating.

As long as you eat slowly and pay attention to your body's signals, it will naturally tell you when to stop and help you eat the right amount. Even if you are served a bowl of Fettuccini Alfredo, which is a notoriously high calorie dish, just take your time and eat slowly. If you do this, you'll probably find you won't even finish your plate, or might only eat half. Just don't be surprised if they say you eat like a bird—but don't worry, that's not a bad thing!

Another challenging time for dieters is the holidays. Whether it's Thanksgiving, Halloween, Christmas, Hanukkah, Kwanza, or even Valentine's Day, these holidays typically include festive celebrations centered around food. With the proper planning you can enjoy your favorite holiday foods without blowing your budget. Don't let these typical diet traps be an excuse for you to go off the deep-end and consume a week's worth of calories in a few days.

The same approach applies when it comes to going on vacation. While on vacation, people find themselves putting on an average of five pounds, if not more. According to WebMD, while on vacation, it's all too easy to abandon everything you know about eating and then return home unable to button your pants. But experts say, it is possible to enjoy your favorite foods and beverages while on vacation without the resulting weight gain.[28]

Even though other people might find themselves gaining weight while on vacation, you don't have to. You can easily maintain your weight, or even lose weight. As long as you have your phone with you, you can track your calories. When you can count your calories, do so, and when you can't, make the lower-calorie choices. You might find counting your calories on vacation too cumbersome, so you can always just focus on eating lower calorie foods and smaller portions.

Vacation is no different than regular life, and don't let it be an excuse to throw everything you've learned out the window. Being that you might be more active on vacation than a regular day at the office; if you are careful about what you eat, you may even find that you lost weight when you get home.

Always strive to stick to your calorie goal while dining out, but if you need to use your "mad money" calories, or make an educated calorie guess, there is no need for concern. Plus, if you listen to your body, it will help you eat the right amount, even when you aren't able to count your calories. Whether you dine out occasionally, or you're on the road and have to eat out most of the time, you can still stick to your goals and lose weight with great success.

CHAPTER 11

THERE IS NO SUCH THING AS CHEATING...ON YOUR DIET

I walk slowly, but I never walk backward.

—Abraham Lincoln

Now you can cheat on your homework and you can cheat on your taxes (just kidding!), but you can't cheat on your diet. That's because as an enlightened dieter, there is no such thing as being on or off your diet. Rather, it's about making choices. You should think of diet enlightenment more as a philosophy than a strict diet that you have to stick to. It's important to understand that you don't need to be perfect all of the time to have weight loss success.

It's really the belief that you can ruin your diet that causes dieters to sabotage their own efforts. The thought is you're either being perfect or you're off your diet, and when you're off your diet, that's a license to binge and overeat. It's this intensity and guilt that causes many dieters to have this overreaction. But that's kind of like going to the mall with a budget, and spending a little more than you planned, and then getting upset and going to the Louis Vuitton store and maxing out your credit cards.

So if you eat a donut and weren't planning on it, there is no reason to feel bad and finish off the entire box. Instead, add the donut to your calorie tracker and adjust your calories for the day accordingly. Even if you happen to go over your calorie budget, don't freak out. Just record what you ate, think about what you could have done differently so you learn from it, and then immediately get back to making smarter choices. A blip here and there will not affect your progress, unless you overreact to it.

Because you can eat anything you want on this program, you're not cheating, you're just making choices. That means there shouldn't be any guilt attached to food. Also, because there is no such thing as cheating on this diet, there are no time-outs so you can restart your diet on Monday. If you eat too many calories, you might slow down your progress, but you're still moving forward. Lastly because you don't have to be perfect all of the time to have success, you don't need to be so hard on yourself. You have to lose the intensity, and in the process you lose the overreaction.

The truth is when you realize that there is no such thing as being off of your diet; it may make you think twice about going off the deep-end. That's because even if you purposely eat an extra 1,000 calories, you still need to record what you ate in your calorie tracker. Besides you're listening to your body, and that means always eating when you're hungry and never eating when you're not. Binge-eating usually has less to do with hunger, and more to do with feeling out of control.

Another thing to keep in mind is that you want to feel great while on your weight loss plan. If you eat too little food, you're going to feel hungry, weak, and miserable. On the other hand, if you overeat and binge, you might enjoy yourself for a fleeting moment, but then after you are going to feel terrible. Not only will you feel ashamed, but physically you're going to be in a lot of discomfort. There should be no reason why you ever feel like you messed up so badly that you want to max out your calories, and cause yourself physical pain.

Since we can't always be perfect, you have to get comfortable with possibly eating something you're not proud of, and not feeling like you cheated or ruined your diet. It might be a good exercise one night to purposely eat a few extra hundred calories over your budget and be okay with it. Remember, one bad meal or even weekend can never ruin weeks or months of progress unless you overreact to it.

That being said, if you're eating lots of delicious food, getting a lot of bang for your calorie, and staying satisfied throughout the day, you should find it very easy to stick to your calorie budget. But if for some reason you go a little over, don't lose your peace of mind. Even if you make a poor choice, there is always a silver lining. It's likely you can learn something and benefit from the situation, so you'll make better choices in the future.

CHAPTER 12

TO SCALE OR NOT TO SCALE...
THAT IS THE QUESTION

The best measure of a man's honesty isn't his income tax return. It's the zero adjust on his bathroom scale.

—Arthur C. Clarke

One of the most common questions that dieters ask is whether or not they should use a bathroom scale to monitor their progress. In fact, there is a big debate in the weight loss community as to whether or not scales should be used. My personal opinion is that while losing weight, you should absolutely use a bathroom scale to weigh yourself. However, you must understand what comes along with using a scale, so you don't fall into the possible frustrations of using one. Regardless of what you decide to do, the reality is that if you're not seeing the bathroom scale move over a period of time, you're probably not losing weight.

Studies show that people who weigh themselves at least once per week lose more weight and keep it off longer than those who don't use a scale. Frankly, I think it comes down to accountability. When you know you're going to be weighing in the next day, or at the end of the week, it gives you a little bit extra motivation to stick to your goal. Plus, monitoring your weight allows you to make adjustments to your program. Overall, when you see how effectively you're losing weight each week, and you have confidence in your plan, it helps you stay on track long-term.

Most importantly, weighing yourself during the course of your weight loss journey allows you to recalculate your daily calorie needs for weight loss. How are you supposed to know how many calories you should consume, if you can't account for your current weight in the formula? While you could estimate that you're losing 1-2 pounds per week, without actually weighing yourself, it's just a guess. You need a scale to accurately determine your current weight. A few pounds up or down—accounting for natural weight fluctuations—won't make a difference, but anything more substantial can affect your calculation.

If you are going to use a scale, it's important to understand a few things. First of all, it's normal for your body weight to fluctuate—usually within one tenth of a pound, and sometimes even up to a few pounds. Changes in your weight can be based on a number of factors including hydration, loss or gain of water weight, and contents of your digestive system, how recent the last meal and bowel movements were.[29] So it's important to account for these natural variances when you weigh-in and monitor your progress, so you don't become discouraged.

If you are consistently sticking to your calorie budget and happen to experience a natural one pound or two weight fluctuation, your number will return to where it should be in a day or so. So if you happen to be up a little on the scale one day, even though you've been sticking to your plan religiously, don't get disheartened. It's likely you're just experiencing a natural weight fluctuation and will return to the correct weight the following day. Slight weight fluctuations can occur from day to day, and even throughout the day itself. That's why you'll notice you usually weigh at least one pound more at night, than you will first thing in the morning. It's important to always weigh yourself with the same conditions each day, but we'll get to that later.

If you have a lot of weight to lose, slight weight fluctuations might not bother you. But, if you're trying to drop those last five pounds, you might feel like every pound, or half a pound counts. It's important to understand natural weight variances, so you don't get frustrated if it happens. Even if you are you just maintaining your weight, it won't be exactly the same every single day. That's especially true if you have a good scale that measures down to the tenth of a pound. For example, over the course of a few days, I might weigh in at 105.5, 106, and 105.8. It's perfectly normal.

The second important factor to consider is that you can only absorb so much weight in one meal. For example, if you were to have a large salty Chinese food dinner and go on the scale the next morning, you could easily be up a few pounds depending on your weight. However, that's likely not actual weight gained. It's probably a combination of water weight from the salt, as well as the food that hasn't left your system yet.

It's important to understand that even if you went over your calorie budget, you didn't gain five pounds in one meal, or ruin all the work you did the week before.

Remember, one bad meal can never sabotage your progress. Sometimes even if you ate the exact correct amount of calories, depending on what you ate, you might be up a pound on the scale. So if you weighed in at 120 pounds yesterday, and after a big salty dinner you weigh 123, don't get upset. I guarantee you, if you stick to your weight loss calorie number over the next day or two, you'll be back to your original number if not less.

The third factor to consider is that, if you're a woman, you may be retaining water during your time of the month. Each woman is different and some women are unaffected, but if you notice you feel bloated or are up a few pounds on the scale, this might be a natural fluctuation. Remember, these are all natural weight fluctuations, and usually account for no more than a pound or two.

Because of these various factors, some experts recommend that dieters stay off the scale because it can be discouraging. They believe that if a dieter does not see progress, or is up a few pounds—due to natural weight fluctuations—they might get frustrated and sabotage their diet or abandon it entirely. While I understand where this thinking comes from, I don't agree with throwing the scales out the window. I believe that with the right knowledge and understanding, dieters can effectively use scales and have more success with them than they would without them.

There are a few things you can do to increase the accuracy of your weigh-ins. Research has shown that digital scales are more accurate than analog. So I recommend investing in a good digital scale—they are not that expensive. You can go to Target, Bed Bath & Beyond, or even order one from Amazon, and get a decent scale for $20-$100. All you really need is a basic digital scale; you don't need all the extra bells and whistles like body fat measurement and memory, unless of course you specifically want that.

If you already have a good scale, make sure you replace the battery if it's older than a few years. Slight weight fluctuations from day to day, or even morning to night are normal. But if you notice that every time you step on the scale, it gives you a completely different number, it may be time to replace the battery, or get a new scale.

To ensure consistency, I recommend that you always weigh yourself first thing in the morning—after you use the bathroom and before you eat anything. I also recommend weighing yourself naked so that you don't have to worry about accounting for clothes. Always do your best to duplicate the weigh-in conditions every time. If it's a digital scale, I usually step on it at least twice in a row to make sure I get the same number.

Unless a scale is broken, or the battery needs to be replaced, a scale doesn't lie. What this means is while you could be up a pound due to a natural weight fluctuation, the scale is not going to tell you that you lost weight, and it's not true.

For the most part, your weight will be accurate. And if you are experiencing a slight fluctuation, it's usually easy to identify why this is happening. So if you happen to eat a really heavy or salty meal, I would recommend not going on the scale the next day. You may want to just wait a day or two, and then go on the scale to get a more accurate number.

If you suspect that your weight is up due to a natural fluctuation, it's important to not let the number on the scale freak you out. If you've ever been on a diet, you know that even one pound up can be extremely frustrating. However, stay the course and continue to weigh yourself over the next few days; if you stick to your calorie budget, your weight will go down guaranteed. Understand that these variances are normal, and know how to spot them, so you don't get discouraged.

Another thing to consider is that when it comes to the scale you don't always lose weight evenly over a week. I remember one particular instance in which I stayed perfectly within my weight loss budget all week, but the scale wouldn't seem to budge. Instead of getting frustrated, I continued the plan because I was confident that I was losing weight. Two days later, I went on the scale again, and I was actually down three more pounds than I even expected. Have faith in the plan and you will see the number you are looking for on the scale.

As we discussed in a previous chapter, you can typically expect to lose on average two pounds per week. If you have a lot of weight to lose and really stick to your weight loss calorie number, you may even lose up to 3 or more pounds per week. If you're near the very end of your weight loss journey , 0.5 to 1 pound per week is a good number. Remember, if you lose it at a slow and healthy rate, you 'll be less likely to gain the weight back.

When it comes to the scale, it's important to be recording your weight and monitoring your progress. You can write this number down in a journal or keep track of it in your calorie tracker program. How often you want to weigh yourself is completely up to you. You can weigh yourself every single day, every other day, twice a week, once a week, or once every two weeks.

Personally, when I was losing weight, I went on the scale every day and found it to be effective. Now that I'm just maintaining my weight, I usually weigh-in only once a week. If you are going to weigh yourself every day, know that there will be slight fluctuations within a tenth of a pound and that's normal. The good thing about weighing yourself everyday is that it keeps you feeling motivated and accountable.

Now if you are the type of person who prefers to wait and see a larger drop on the scale than you could weigh yourself once a week or every other week. If you are going to do this, I recommend weighing yourself two days in a row to allow for more accuracy. Also, I'd recommend weighing in on a Friday morning before the weekend for obvious reasons. My recommendtion is to go on the scale every day, but how often you want to weigh yourself is completely up to you. This should not be stressful and it should be something you look forward to, especially as you 're watching the number on the scale go down.

Overall, don't spend too much time obsessing about tiny fluctuations. At most, weight fluctuations are typically within a pound or two and usually correct themselves within a few days. If for some reason, you are not losing weight on the scale over a longer period of time, then you may want to make some adjustments. Perhaps you're overestimating your workout calories. Or if you are consistently using your "mad money" calories you may want to cut down on those. In my experience, as long as you are cognizant about measuring your food calories and workout calories, that won't be an issue.

In addition to the scale, there are other ways that will help encourage you that you've lost weight. Seeing how your clothes fit after a month of being on the plan can be a great way to judge weight loss. For example, if you dropped 10 pounds, you'll have a lot more room in your pants. If you are losing weight, you will notice that your clothes fit differently!

Being that you see yourself in the mirror every day, it's unlikely that you'll notice a difference in your appearance at first. But trust me people around you will start to notice. As you start dropping pounds, people might start coming up to you, and asking if you've lost weight. There's nothing better for your diet morale than someone asking if you've lost weight or telling you how fantastic you look.

Now if you're a guy, you might not care so much about the number on the scale—at least the way us women do. You may be just thinking about losing the spare tire, getting rid of your gut, or eliminating the pudge. So in addition to the scale, another thing you can do to help gauge your progress is to have your body fat measured by a physician or personal trainer. But again, the scale doesn't lie. If you legitimately lost weight, your clothes will feel much looser, your body fat will be down, and you will weigh less on the scale.

One last thing that I need to touch on when it comes to the scale is the whole muscle versus fat issue. Yes, muscle does weigh more than fat. However, people typically overestimate how much muscle weight they gain by starting a cardio program and getting toned. With the exception of professional athletes and body builders, you don't need to worry about it offsetting your weight loss on the scale.

For my serious weight lifters, if you lifted weights prior to starting this diet and keep it up, then you don't need to worry about gaining muscle weight as you're just maintaining. On the other hand, if you're purposely trying to gain a certain amount of muscle weight while losing weight, you can work with a fitness professional to help determine that amount.

According to the article titled the "Weight Loss Plateau Myth: Muscle Weighs More Than Fat?" The average natural male who is past the beginner stage of weight lifting and doing everything right, might gain 0.25 lb of muscle per week under the best possible circumstances. The average female fitting the same description might gain half of that. On the other hand, the average person with an average amount of fat to lose will typically lose it at rate of 1-2lbs per week without a problem."[30]

The author continues to point out that, "So the clear message here is that in *most* of the cases where you see *no* weight loss for an *extended* period of time and think it's because muscle weighs more than fat and you are really losing fat but just simultaneously gaining an equal amount of muscle at an equal rate—you're probably wrong. And by probably, I mean you're wrong 99 percent of the time."[31]

It is unlikely that weight lifting will interfere with your weight loss on the scale, especially if you're like most people and just looking to tone up. Plus, when we're talking about best possible circumstances, picture Arnold Schwarzenegger in Pumping Iron. If that reference is lost on you, picture Vin Diesel or Dwayne "The Rock" Johnson. But in all seriousness, if you're trying to add muscle weight, the most you can typically gain in one year is roughly 13 pounds if you are a man and 6.5 pounds if you are a woman.

If you are just toning up and not bulking up, then do not worry about muscle weight affecting your weight loss. Plus, when you gain muscle, you burn more calories at a resting rate. Personally, after I got down to my my goal weight, I started working out more and lifting weights to tone up, and my weight stayed exactly the same.

When it comes to the scale, you might be wondering what a good weight is for you. Trust me once you start seeing how efficiently you drop the weight, you'll understand why it's important to determine an ideal weight. If you are looking for some information or direction on what's a healthy weight range for you, there are plenty of free resources available online.

You can check out the nifty Ideal Body Weight Calculator available on www.freedieting.com. This calculator uses your gender, height, and body frame (small, medium, or large) to calculate an estimated ideal weight range.

In order to determine your body frame, you can do a simple test. Grip your wrist using your thumb and middle finger. If your finger and thumb don't touch you have a large frame. If your finger and thumb just touch or barely touch you have a medium frame. If your finger and thumb easily touch or overlap you have a small frame. Use the above calculator to see what your recommended weight range is.

For example, I'm 5'2" and have a small frame; it says my ideal weight range is between 102 and 106. Really, what this means is that that the lowest I can go down to without becoming underweight is 102. Personally, I like to split the difference and use 105 as my ideal weight. While I enjoy being slim, it's very important to stay at a healthy weight range. If you are overweight or underweight it puts you at risk for many health issues.

You can also use a BMI calculator to see what category your current weight and ideal weight fall into: underweight, normal weight, overweight, moderately obese, or severely obese. Body Mass Index (BMI) is a number calculated from a person's weight and height; it does not account for gender. While men and women distribute and carry weight differently, a BMI calculator can still help to make sure you don't fall underweight or overweight.

Here is a list of free online BMI calculators you can use:

1. Mayo Clinic BMI Calculator:
    www.mayoclinic.org/diseases-conditions/obesity/in-depth/bmi-calculator/itt-20084938

2. LiveStrong BMI Calculator:
    www.livestrong.com/tools/body-mass-calculator

3. Free Dieting BMI Calculator:
    www.freedieting.com/bmi-calculator

Keep in mind that any BMI or Idea Body Weight Calculator should only be used as a reference. It doesn't reflect your individual body composition. You can always check with your physician to make sure you are at a healthy weight. As long as you are in a healthy weight range, if you like a little extra junk in your trunk, by all means go for it. Ultimately, how much you want to weigh should be completely up to you.

So when it comes to that famous question, "To Scale or Not to Scale?" my answer is definitely yes! I highly recommend using a bathroom scale to help monitor your weight loss and progress. But remember, you must understand what goes along with using one, so that it doesn't drive you crazy.

Using a bathroom scale is also especially useful once you get down to your goal weight. While maintaining your weight, getting on the scale once a week is a good way to make sure you don't gain the weight back. If you happen to gain a little weight around the holidays, it's much easier to take off a few pounds than to wake up one day and realize you put on 20 pounds. Now with the diet enlightenment approach, you'll be way less likely to put weight back on because you've learned how to lose weight while eating the types of foods you like to eat. However, being an enlightened dieter is not just about losing weight, it is about maintining it as well. Going on the scale periodically is a good way to make sure you are staying on track. Make peace with the scale, and it can be a great tool that will help you succeed

CHAPTER 13
YOUR DIET JOURNEY

Even a journey of a thousand miles begins with
a single step.

—Lao Tzu

Now that you have all of the knowledge and tools
you need, you can begin your diet journey. I like
to think of this journey as a cross-country train with a
series of stops. It's no different than getting on a train
from Chicago to Los Angeles. Don't get off at Kansas
City or Topeka; stay the course, stay on track, and you
will get to your destination guaranteed.

Sticking with this analogy, you're pretty much on
an express train because as an enlightened dieter you
are dieting efficiently. Nevertheless, even express trains
have stops and checkpoints along the way. In this
chapter, I want to help walk you through the first week,
first weekend, first event, and first few months, so you
stay motivated and on track.

Remember, this is meant to be a natural and smooth
journey. As the weeks go by, you will constantly be
learning more, getting more creative, and becoming
more confident. Be patient with yourself and stay the
course. The longer you do it, the easier it will become.

By the time you lose all the weight, you'll be wondering how you could have ever tried any other weight loss plan. So pack your bags and get on board. Welcome to the diet enlightenment journey.

When it comes to starting your diet journey, what day of the week you want to begin is completely up to you. I recommend starting on a Monday because it represents the beginning of the week. However, you can start your diet any day you want.

Whatever day you do choose to start, keep in mind that you will actually start preparing for it the day before. For example, if you are going to start this program on a Wednesday then on Tuesday morning you should go on the scale to check your weight, figure out how many calories you get, and start thinking about and planning your meals for the next day.

The day before you start your diet is an opportunity to think about what foods you like and want to eat. It's also an opportunity to do some research and consider what foods you can incorporate that are low in calories and high in bulk; just make sure it's something you'll enjoy. Remember what you learned in chapter 8 about the art of choosing what you eat, and how to get more bang for your calorie.

While you could spend your first few days eating nothing but high-calorie junk food, the point of this diet is to be able to eat a lot of food, so you're not feeling hungry. It's one thing to stick within your calorie budget, but another thing to do so easily and effortlessly. So make sure to try and incorporate lots of high-bulk, low-calorie options into your plan. If you're doing this diet right, it shouldn't even feel like a typical diet.

As you're planning what you are going to eat, think about whether you will cook your meals at home, go out to eat at a restaurant, or do a combination of both. Come up with a tentative meal plan that you feel good about and will keep you satisfied. Have a lot of fun with this and be creative.

Hands down, one of the most important and crucial recommendations that I will give you on this program is to plan out your meals ahead of time —specifically plan our your meals for the next day the night before in your calorie tracker or journal. If you want to do this program right, this is a must! So plan out your day of meals ahead of time, then if what you eat changes, you can adjust your meals and calories for the rest of the day accordingly. It's good to think about and plan what you are going to eat ahead of time, but also have flexibility if it changes.

For those of you who've never counted calories, or kept track of what you consumed, this will be a totally new habit. But just like any habit, before long it'll be second nature. Regardless of what you eat and how often you eat, make sure you write down what you consume every single day. It's important to start developing this habit of recording what you eat. You will have so much more success if you accurately record what you eat rather than just trying to remember it in your head.

On your first official day of your diet, it's important to weigh yourself that morning, record your weight, and double check your formula to confirm your calories.

In the beginning of this diet, my recommendation is to make it as convenient for yourself as possible. Now if you are a chef or passionate about cooking, then you may dive right into cooking delicious, low-calorie recipes for your favorite foods. But, if you are are like most people, you may not feel like you have time to do that at first. You might have a hectic work schedule, are still in school, or are busy with kids. Or maybe due to your job, you are always on the road and need to eat out.

Regardless, if you aren't able to make your meals at home or you do not have the time, I recommend identifying a few restaurants that list their nutritional information online and you can grab for lunch or dinner. It should be easy and convenient, and most of all filling and delicious. As an example, a turkey sub from Subway or a burrito bowl from Chipotle. At either of these restaurants it's easy to find high density, low calorie options that fit within your calorie budget for that meal. You can also couple that with finding low-calorie but delicious snacks to fill in the gaps. It's a very easy and convenient way to kick-start your first week.

If you are going to cook at home, you might want to focus on cooking meals for one. What that means is, even if you need to cook dinner for your family, you could prepare something separate for yourself. The great thing about this diet is that you can customize it to accommodate your schedule. You can always start simple and basic, and get more creative with time. Once you really get the hang of it, you'll find you can almost always create a lower calorie version of your favorite dish.

To give you an example, when I first put my dad on this diet, he was a busy doctor and didn't have time to prepare his meals at home; or at least he didn't think he did. He literally went to Subway for lunch the entire first two weeks. Granted it worked great for him, and he lost six pounds in those first two weeks. But thankfully by the third week, I was able to convince him to start incorporating other restaurants and to start making more meals at home.

What he didn't realize at the time was when you prepare food yourself you can be so much more creative. I remember taking him to the grocery store and walking down every single aisle. I helped him pick out foods that he liked that could deliver a lot of bang for the calorie. Trust me— there is a heck of a lot of food out there that is delicious, low-calorie, and satisfying. It was an eye opening experience for him. He was shocked to find that even when it came to his favorite foods, there were many lower-calorie alternatives available.

Down the road you'll be a pro at essentially eating whatever you want; however, for the first week, I recommend focusing on filling but low calorie items, so you're eating a lot of food. Remember, when you're full and satisfied you'll feel good, and feeling good makes dieting easy.

In addition to figuring out what you're going to eat, you'll want to think about how you're going to split up your calories. For example, I'm rarely hungry in the morning, so I like to have a light breakfast and eat the majority of my calories for lunch and dinne. My husband, on the other hand, is the complete opposite and likes to consume the majority of his calories earlier in the day.

If you're not sure how you want to split up your calories, I suggest eating three square meals per day and filling in the gaps with low-calorie snacks if you get hungry. Most importantly, you should be listening to your body; that is, eating whenever you're legitimately hungry and never eating when you are not hungry . As you continue through your diet journey, you 'll learn what works the best for you.

Another good suggestion when starting out is to save at least 50-100 calories for a post-dinner snack. This way if you eat dinner early at 5:30pm or 6pm, you are not done for the rest of the day, and can still have something a little later to look forward to. I personally try not to eat anything past 7pm, but calories are still calories regardless of what time you consume them at. I have just noticed that my willpower falls off a proverbial cliff later at night so I try to avoid the kitchen all together.

Overall during your first week, remember the following points: keep your meals convenient; make sure you're enjoying the food you eat; try to eat foods that are lower in calories and higher in volume; and make sure you don't let yourself go hungry. Also, if you really want something that's higher in calories, figure out a way to work it into your budget, so you don't feel like you're denying yourself. Whether you want to eat out for all of your meals, or make every meal from scratch, the choice is up to you.

The first stop on your diet journey is typically the first weekend. I consider this a stop or checkpoint because weekends can be challenging for some people.

But just because there is a stop there, don't get off the train. When it comes to diets, many find themselves being perfect Monday through Friday, and then going off the deep-end on the weekend. However, this is usually because they're sticking to a plan during the week that leaves them hungry and bereft of their favorite food. However, as an enlightened dieter you shouldn't have this problem.

Weekends are your time to explore and be creative. Try cooking new low-calorie recipes for your favorite dishes, or practice eating out successfully. If you can, strive to find restaurants that list their nutritional information online so it's even easier. Whether you're dining out at restaurants or eating at home, with the proper planning you should have no problem sticking to your calorie budget. And remember, just because you are off from work, doesn't mean you're off from recording what you eat.

When it comes to weekends, you can always choose to use your "mad money" or additional calories. But, you may find that you don't even need to. With the extra free time to work-out and plan your meals, you may find weekends even easier than weekdays. As long as you're eating great food and keeping yourself full and satisfied, sticking to your plan will feel easy and effortless.

Once you've made it past your first full week, including weekend, it's going to get easier. You've laid a good foundation and will find the process more enjoyable. If you haven't already done so, now is the time to start expanding the restaurants you can go to, and introducing more foods to your diet. Go to the grocery store, the local market, and continue to look for new and delicious foods to incorporate. You may find that you like to eat the same things every day, but with a little research you also might find something even better and for fewer calories.

The next stop along the way will likely be your first event. It might be a wedding, a party, or simply eating out at someone's house. It will be an instance in which you can't necessarily count your calories, and will need to consciously make low-calorie choices. Remember, if 95 percent of the time you can eat whatever you want and count your calories, then the few times you can't, it's totally reasonable to focus on low-calorie options or small portions on these occasions. Again, this is an opportunity to make smart decisions, listen to your body, and eat like a thin person.

Another important stop, or checkpoint along the way is your one-month mark. They say if you can stick to something for twenty-one days, it then becomes a habit. I'm not sure if that's true, but I do know after a month of being on this plan, you will look and feel amazing. You should feel very proud of yourself for reaching the one-month mark. Even if you had to use your "mad money" at times or weren't perfect one day, you still stayed the course.

As the weeks and months go by, remember what we talked about in Chapter 11. You don't have to be perfect during this journey to have success. While this plan should be very easy to stick to, if you happen to go over your maintenance number one day, don't overreact and worry that you sabotaged your progress. In fact, your body can only absorb a certain amount of weight per day. While you shouldn't be overeating, if you eat too much one night, just immediately get back on track, and it won't even make a difference in the long run.

Think of it like being on a train, and getting up to go sit in the cart behind you. Unless you physically get off the train, you're still on track and it's not going to affect your arrival. Now if you overreact and metaphorically jump off the train, then sure it will certainly slow down your progress. But one bad meal or even weekend will never hurt your diet in the long run as long as you always get back on track.

Throughout your journey, remember to weigh yourself each week so you can recalculate your weight loss number calorie needs. It's a very satisfying feeling to get on that scale and watch the number to continue to drop. Keep track of your progress, and record your weigh-ins in your calorie tracker or journal.

As you start losing weight, not only will you be getting thinner, but also your stomach will slowly shrink, and it will take less food to fill you up. Plus, you should notice that when you listen to your body's needs and eat accordingly, you feel fantastic. To the contrary, overfeeding your body or underfeeding it will make you feel like crap both physically and mentally. And enlightened dieters know better than this. Choose the path of least resistance and feel good.

As the months go by, you'll start noticing significant weight loss. In addition to weighing less on the scale, your clothes will feel looser and you might notice people making comments about how great you look.

You'll also have much more energy, and notice you're less preoccupied with food.

While you are losing weight steadily, some of you might get antsy because you want to have lost everything by now. The Sistine Chapel wasn't painted in one day, and you can't lose 40 pounds in two weeks. But you are losing weight as quickly and efficiently as possible while still staying healthy. Some of you might feel the urge to eat less calories, or do something extreme, but stick to the plan.

Enjoy yourself while you are losing the weight. Don't let yourself get impatient. This diet works! While hopefully you're eating a lot of low-calorie, high-bulk items to keep you full, you're also eating anything you want. If you want to eat a slice of birthday cake for a special occasion, fit it into your budget. If your family is going out for pizza, that's perfectly okay. If you really want that Baby Ruth candy bar, make it work. It's all about having a balance, and not depriving yourself. When things are no longer off-limits, they start to lose their intensity and allure.

Your second to the last stop on this journey is your last five pounds. Metaphorically, you're pulling into the station and the train starts to slow down. Don't be discouraged if you only lose between 0.5 and 1 pound per week during this last part of your diet. Continue to stay on track and you will reach your dream weight guaranteed.

The last stop on the train is your dream weight—your final destination. The great thing about this achievement is not only do you look and feel great, but you now know that you'll always have control over your weight. In the next chapter, we will discuss how to maintain your weight loss easily. It is just as important to master diet maintenance as it is to lose the weight.

CHAPTER 14
DIET MAINTENANCE

If you have planted a tree you must water it too.

—Indian proverb

Whether your diet journey took a few weeks, a few months, or even a full year, you've now achieved your dream weight. And that is certainly something to be proud of! To quote Nelson Mandela, "It always seems impossible until it's done." Isn't that the truth! But now that you've achieved your goal, it's important to learn how to maintain it. What's the point of losing weight, if you're just going to gain it back? Diet enlightenment is just as much about maintaining your weight loss as it is about losing it.

The good news is that it's even easier to maintain your weight than it is to lose it. Because you lost weight eating the foods you like, learned how to count calories and get more bang for your calories, learned how to listen to your body, and unlearned destructive emotional eating habits —you've essentially programmed yourself for long-term success. Plus, maintenance is easier than weight loss, simply because you get more calories.

When the time comes to figure out your daily calorie needs for weight maintenance, you'll use the same online calculator you used before. You've already done the calculation to figure out your daily calorie needs—the difference is you won't be subtracting the 20 percent for weight loss, or essentially looing at the weight loss number. Now you're in maintenance.

Here is the link to the online calculator that I provided in Chapter 6. Use it to determine your daily calorie needs for maintenance:

www.freedieting.com/calorie-calculator

For example, if you're a thirty year old female, standing five foot five, and weighing 115 pounds, you'll get roughly 1500 calories per day to maintain your current weight. That's an additional 300 calories from when you were losing weight! In another example, if you're a thirty year old male, standing five foot ten, and weighing 160 pounds, you'll get roughly 2,000 calories for maintenance; that's an additional 400 calories!

As you can see, depending on your individual factors, you'll get approximately between 300-400 additional calories when transitioning to maintenance. That doesn't even account for the extra calories you can add for exercise. If you happen to go a little under or a little over your maintenance number that's fine, but try to consistently stay as close to that number as possible. And yes in this case, it's always better to go a little under than over. Being that during the last few weeks of your weight loss journey, you probably got very good at sticking to your weight loss calorie number—now getting all of these additional calories should be super easy!

In fact, when I first made the transition from daily calorie needs for weight loss to maintenance, I didn't even know what to do with all those extra calories. Trust me; it's a good problem to have.

During maintenance, it's important to continue to weigh yourself on the scale each week. Not only does it continue to make you feel accountable, but also, it'll make sure you keep the weight off. If for some reason you notice you put on an extra few pounds, and it's not a natural weight fluctuation, then you can just figure out your weight loss calorie number and get back to your ideal weight. Or if you happen to get pregnant, you can happily put on the healthy recommended amount of weight, and know that you can easily get it off in the future.

As time goes on, make sure you continue to recalculate your maintenance number because the older you get, the less calories you need. So many people complain that they put on weight as they age because their metabolism slows down. That type of thinking makes it seem like weight control is out of your hands. In reality, as long as you recalculate your maintenance number, which factors in your age, you will always consume the right amount of calories.

A diet maintenance should be an easy and enjoyable time. It should be an overwhelming sense of peace. Possibly for the first time in your life, dieting isn't an issue for you. Plus, have fun with it and continue to explore new lower calorie, high bulk recipes, foods, and menu items to give you even more satisfaction.

Eventually you might come to a point where you've lost the weight and maintained it for a long enough time and don't want to count your calories all of the time. Because you've gotten used to eating smaller portions, stopping when you're full, knowing which items will keep you satisfied and basically eating like a thin person, you should be able to have great success with just listening to your body. That's how naturally thin people stay thin without counting their calories.

Personally, I still like to count my calories and always will because I find it incredibly easy and I like sticking to a budget—whether it's financial or caloric. You might find this analogy strange, but you don't stop having a budget when you get a big raise or if you become a millionaire— or you'll end up in debt or broke. Let that sink in for a second. Is it really that far of a stretch to budget, plan, and watch your calories? Having a set plan or budget, even if it's just to maintain your weight, is a good way to make sure you stay on track.

I said it earlier and I'll say it again —counting your calories is a very small price to pay to get to maintain your perfect weight and eat what you like. Being able to design my day with my favorite foods within a budget is strangely rewarding. Plus, I've been doing it for so long now that it's truly like second nature. Perhaps, you'll plan and monitor your calories during the week, and choose not to do so on the weekends. You'll discover what works best for you after you've lost the weight and it comes time to maintain it.

Really what I think makes this dieting approach different and so special is that you lose the weight the same exact way you maintain it. So even if you've lost weight in the past on other diets, but put the weight back on, you won't have that same problem this time. Master the art of weight loss and you'll master diet maintenance.

CHAPTER 15
FOOD FOR THOUGHT

Nobody can bring you peace, but yourself.

—Ralph Waldo Emerson

Throughout your journey, I encourage you to reread this book or sections of this book. It will help remind you that not only are you monitoring your calories, but also you're changing the way you think and feel about food. Keep in mind that while I do refer to this as a diet, it's really a paradigm shift. As an enlightened dieter, it's not just about calories and pounds; it's about finding peace of mind.

The truth is that wanting and struggling to lose weight, can be just as much of a burden as being overweight. For those of you who've struggled with weight issues for most of your lives, and have tried everything else, diet enlightenment can be your salvation. It's interesting that weight loss, something that can cause so much frustration, is the most easily accomplished with ease.

This diet isn't about willpower, sacrifice, or discipline; it's about enthusiasm, creativity, planning, and attention to detail. It's not about trying to control hunger; it's about making sure you stay satisfied, so losing weight is easy. It's definitely not about quick results and gimmicks; it's about sound, scientific research that works. Lastly, it's not about struggle; it's about the path of least resistance.

During your journey, you don't even need to think about weight loss that much; it's happening behind the scenes. Instead, focus on designing delicious meals, and how you will feel when you reach your dream weight. It might mean fitting into your jeans from high school, making a difference in your dating life, going off medication, or staying alive longer for your kids. Or it may just mean realizing that you don't have to settle for being overweight, and that you can truly achieve anything your heart desires.

Becoming an enlightened dieter is about seeing through the clutter and nonsense. It's about discovering the truth and embracing its simplicity, so you can achieve permanent weight loss. When you do finally lose the weight and become awakened, you'll laugh because it truly is so simple. Master the art of weight loss and maintenance, and you'll break the cycle and be free.

ENDNOTES

1   The Real Cause of the Global Obesity Epidemic (March 20, 2012) http://investmentwatchblog.com/the-real-cause-of-the-global-obesity-epidemic-2/

2   American Journal of Preventitive Medicine. Obesity and Severe Obseity Forecasts Through 2030. Volume 42, Issue 6, P563-570, June 1, 2012. https://www.ajpmonline.org/article/S%200749-3797(12%20)00146-8/fulltext

3   The New England Journal of Medicine. "Comparison of Weight-Loss Diets with Different Compositions of Fat, Protein, and Carbohydrates." 2009.

4   Uncovering the Atkins Diet Secret." *BBC News*. BBC, 21 Jan. 2004. Web. 16 Apr. 2012. http://news.bbc.co.uk/2/hi/health/3416637.stm.

5   "The Atkins Diet transcript" http://www.bbc.co.uk/science/horizon/2004/atkinstrans.shtml

6   "Dieticians Warn of Low-Carbo Diet Dangers". http://www.atkinsexposed.org/atkins/97/dietitians_warn_of_low-carbo_diet_dangers.htm

7   The World's Most Dangerous Diets. http://www.weightcritic.com/dangerous_diets.html

8 "HCG Diet Dangers: Is Fast Weight Loss Worth the Risk?" Angela Haupt. March 14, 2011. < http://health.usnews.com/health-news/diet-fitness/diet/articles/2011/03/14/hcg-diet-dangers-is-fast-weight-loss-worth-the-risk>

9 http://www.huffingtonpost.com/2012/04/18/k-e-diet-does-it-work_n_1432790.html

10 New England Journal of Medicine (February 23, 2013) Primary Prevention of Cardiovascular Disease with a Mediterranean Diet (http://www.nejm.org/doi/full/10.1056/NEJMoa1200303?query=OF&)

11 Mayo Clinic article (http://www.mayoclinic.com/health/mediterranean-diet/CL00011)

12 http://www.time.com/time/magazine/article/0,9171,1914974,00.html TIME Magazine

13 http://www.livestrong.com/article/348-smart-shopping-gym-memberships/ LIVESTRONG.com

14 http://well.blogs.nytimes.com/2009/11/04/phys-ed-why-doesnt-exercise-lead-to-weight-loss/

15 http://well.blogs.nytimes.com/2009/11/04/phys-ed-why-doesnt-exercise-lead-to-weight-loss/

16 http://www.merriam-webster.com/dictionary/calorie

17 http://www.livestrong.com/article/178764-caloric-intake-formula/

18 http://www.freedieting.com/tools/calories_burned.htm

19 Why Don't Wild Animals Get Fat. http://the guycancook.com/blog/2010/10/28/why-dont-wild-animals-get-fat/

20 Why Don't Wild Animals Get Fat. http://theguy cancook.com/blog/2010/10/28/why-dont-wild-animals-get-fat/

21 Why Don't Wild Animals Get Fat. http://theguycancook.com/blog/2010/10/28/why-dont-wild-animals-get-fat/

22 Why Don't Wild Animals Get Fat. http://theguycancook.com/blog/2010/10/28/why-dont-wild-animals-get-fat/

23 http://www.dummies.com/how-to/content/id-77555.html

24 http://www.fda.gov/Food/LabelingNutrition/ucm248732.htm

25 http://www.webmd.com/diet/features/low-calorie-cocktails

26 http://www.webmd.com/diet/features/avoid-vacation-weight-gain-5-simple-rules

27 http://www.fittothecorebymargie.com/qabffmweighing.html

28 http://www.aworkoutroutine.com/weight-loss-plateau-myth-muscle-weighs-more-than-fat/

29 http://www.aworkoutroutine.com/weight-loss-plateau-myth-muscle-weighs-more-than-fat/

Made in the USA
Middletown, DE
11 December 2022

18005773R00097